ATKINS DIET FOR BEGINNERS 2021:

THE ULTIMATE GUIDE TO LIVING A LOW-CARB LIFESTYLE.

THE BIBLE OF RECIPES ON ATKINS DIET.
(IN 20 MINUTES OR LESS)

AUTHOR:
CHARLOTTE CONLAN

TABLE OF CONTENTS

THE ATKINS DIET
BRIEF HISTORY

The founder and father of low-carb diets, Robert Atkins may not have been the first to harness the appeal of carb-free, but he was certainly the first to bring the concept to the mainstream dieting public.

In 1963, American physician and cardiologist Robert Atkins came across a study published by Dr. Alfred W. Pennington. His research explored the theory that cutting starch and sugar from the diet could lead to significant weight loss. Putting the pound-shedding theory to the test, Atkins shrunk his own bulk and adapted the findings into the diet and formidable brand we know today.

The Atkins diet is a low-carb diet, usually recommended for weight loss.

Proponents of this diet claim that you can lose weight while eating as much protein and fat as you want, as long as you avoid foods high in carbs.

Studies have shown that low-carb diets without the need of calorie counting, are effective for weight loss and can lead to various health improvements.

The Atkins diet was originally promoted by the physician Dr. Robert C. Atkins, who wrote a best-selling book about it in 1972.

Since then, the Atkins diet has been popular all over the world with many more books having been written.

The diet was originally considered unhealthy and demonized by the mainstream health authorities, mostly due to its high saturated fat content. However, new studies suggest that saturated fat is harmless. Since then, the diet has been studied thoroughly and shown to lead to greater weight loss and greater improvements in blood sugar, "good" HDL cholesterol, triglycerides and other health markers than low-fat diets.

Despite being high in fat, it does not raise "bad" LDL cholesterol on average, though this does happen in a subset of individuals.

The main reason why low-carb diets are so

effective for weight loss is that a reduction in carbs and increased protein intake lead to reduced appetite, making you eat fewer calories without having to think about it.

The Atkins diet was based on Atkins' belief that it's the carbs in our diets which are responsible for our weight gain and that by eating more protein,so we can switch on the "satiated" trigger, which helps us control our appetite. For this reason strict limits are put on carbs especially during the initial weight loss stage, but unlike most other diets there are no restrictions on the amount of fat you can eat. Unsurprisingly, it's during this initial phase that most weight loss is achieved, although much of this is thought to be because of the loss of glycogen stores combined with water, and this is easily re-gained once carbs are re-introduced.

The plan encourages dieters to cut out processed, refined carbs as well as alcohol but allows the inclusion of red meat, butter, cream and cheese. The only fat Atkins suggests you avoid are the man-made trans fats typically found in spreads and processed foods. These trans fats have been linked to clogged arteries and an increased risk of heart disease and stroke.

Enjoying some fat in a healthy, balanced diet is important because it help promote our absorption of fat soluble vitamins like vitamin A, D, E and K, and certain fats are essential to health. These essential omega fats are needed in the diet for the manufacture of hormones and for a healthy nervous system.

More recent evidence is also suggesting that the saturated fat in dairy foods may be less harmful than we once thought. However, although Atkins places no limit on saturates, public health advice remains that we should limit our consumption to 20g of saturates daily. Choosing lower fat animal products like poultry, fish and lean cuts of pork would help towards this. In order to achieve your 5-a-day, any follower of the Atkins diet needs to understand which fruit and vegetable are low carb, so it's important to understand what is a starchy veg (those restricted by the diet) and those which are non-starchy (those which can be included). Good choices of non-starchy veg would be courgette, cucumber and leafy greens like spinach. Low carb fruits would include avocado and olives. Eating a wide range of fruit and veg not only allows us to get plenty of vitamins and fibre but also means we benefit from protective plant compounds like flavonoids and carotenoids which help fight heart disease, certain cancers and may help delay the signs of aging. Most health professionals believe that cutting out major food groups may be detrimental to long term health and in particular a high protein diet, like Atkins, if followed consistently over a long term may have an adverse effect on areas such as bone health, as well as renal function for those with an existing kidney condition.

THE ATKINS DIET

The Atkins diet is similar to a ketogenic diet as both emphasise the consumption of fat and protein but severely restrict carbohydrates. The body will turn to glycogen stores (carbohydrates) for energy first if supplies are plentiful. Ketogenic diets essentially force the body to switch from burning carbohydrates for energy to burning fat. This often has the desirable effect of weight loss, though high levels of ketones in the body can be problematic and may lead to a state known as ketosis.

The Atkins diet aims to help a person lose weight by limiting carbohydrates and controlling insulin levels. Dieters can eat as much fat and protein as they want.

The Atkins diet is designed to reduce carbohydrate intake significantly. The Atkins Diet has four core principles:

- to lose weight
- to maintain weight loss
- to achieve good health

- to lay a permanent foundation for disease prevention

The main reason for weight gain is the consumption of refined carbohydrates, or carbs, especially sugar, high fructose corn syrup, and flour.

When a person follows the Atkins Diet, their body's metabolism switches from burning glucose, or sugar, as fuel to burning stored body fat. This switch is called ketosis.

When glucose levels are low, insulin levels are also low, and ketosis occurs. In other words, when glucose levels are low, the body switches to using its fat stores, as well as dietary fat, for energy. In theory, this can help a person lose body fat and weight.

Before a person eats, their glucose levels are low, so their insulin levels are also low. When that person eats, their glucose levels rise, and the body produces more insulin to help it use glucose.

The glycemic index (GI) is a scale that ranks carbohydrates, or carbs, from 0 to 100, depending on how quickly they increase blood sugar levels after consumption, and by how much.

Refined carbs, such as white bread and candy, contain high levels of glucose. These foods have high GI scores, as their carbs enter the blood rapidly, causing a glucose spike.

Other types of carbs, such as beans, do not affect blood glucose levels so quickly or severely. They have a low glycemic load and score lower on the glycemic index.

Net carbs are the total carbs minus fiber and sugar alcohols. Sugar alcohols have a minimal effect on blood sugar levels. According to Dr. Atkins, the best carbs are those with a low glycemic load.

Fruits and grains are high in carbs, and a person on the Atkins diet restricts these, especially in the early stages. However, these foods are also good sources of vitamins, minerals, fiber, and antioxidants.

To make up for the lack of nutrient-rich foods, the Atkins diet encourages people to use vitamin and mineral supplements.

The Atkins diet may help a person lose weight. For many, losing weight will also reduce the risk of type 2 diabetes, cardiovascular disease, and other aspects of metabolic syndrome.

While a low carb approach may not work or be sustainable for everyone, clinical trials show that the Atkins diet results in similar or greater weight loss in those following it for at least 12 months compared to other options, such as the Mediterranean or DASH diets.

People who use medication for diabetes, cardiovascular disease, and other conditions should not stop taking these when they follow this or any other diet.

USING THE FAT IN THE BODY

If there is minimal carbs intake via the diet, ketosis will occur. During ketosis, the body will breakdown fat stores in the cells, resulting in the creation of ketones. These ketones then become available for the body to use as energy.

The Atkins diet is a low carb diet where the body burns more calories than on other diets because ketosis occurs. It is a kind of ketogenic diet, though protein intake is typically higher, and fat is lower in comparison to a traditional ketogenic diet.

HOW ATKINS DIET WORKS

THE ATKINS DIET: GETTING STARTED, STAYING FOCUSED

The Atkins Diet is an organized program for achieving permanent weight control through the intelligent consumption of carbohydrates. And there's more than weight loss at stake here: what really matters is your overall health and well being. In fact, many people who don't need to lose weight choose to follow the Atkins because of all the health benefits it provides.

Atkins is a four-phase lifetime eating plan that helps you:

- Achieve a carbohydrate awareness regarding quality and quantity of carbohydrates consumed
- Learn your individual threshold for carbohydrate consumption
- Incorporate vitamin and mineral supplementation and regular exercise

Here's what else you need to know about Atkins:

- Though certain guidelines must be followed, the Atkins is flexible, with a wide variety of choices to suit a variety of eating preferences and lifestyles.
- Atkins is not a one-size-fits-all approach—it is a customized eating plan that you will match to your unique metabolism. By learning your individual threshold for carbohydrate consumption, you can reach your ideal goal weight and stay there—without hunger pangs or feelings of deprivation.

THE FOUR PRINCIPLES OF ATKINS DIET

Atkins is based on four core principles, all backed by solid scientific research:

• **Weight loss**

• **Weight maintenance**

• **Good health and well-being**

• **Disease prevention**

THE FOUR PRINCIPLES

Let's take a closer look at the four principles of Atkins:

• **Weight Loss:** Both men and women who follow Atkins readily lose pounds and inches. If you're one of the very few who has a truly hard-core metabolic resistance to weight loss, there are ways to overcome the barriers that prevent a successful outcome.

• **Weight Maintenance:** Most low-fat, low-calorie diets may fail for one reason: hunger. Although many people can tolerate hunger for a while, very few can tolerate it for a lifetime. When you do Atkins, you feel satisfied by the foods you eat; you gradually find your effective individual level of carbohydrate intake, which is the tool that allows you to maintain a healthy weight for a lifetime.

• **Good Health and Well-Being:** With Atkins, you'll meet your nutritional needs by eating healthy, wholesome foods and omitting junk food. You'll find that this results in less fatigue—not just because you're losing pounds, but also because you will stabilize your blood sugar. When you do Atkins, you start feeling good long before they reach your goal weight.

• **Disease Prevention:** By following an individualized controlled-carbohydrate nutritional approach that results in lower insulin production, people at high risk for chronic illnesses such as cardiovascular disease, hypertension and diabetes will see a marked improvement in their health.

BENEFITS OF THE ATKINS DIET

The Atkins diet is becoming very popular nowadays and it has developed very many competitors who provide diets with similar principles. It is basically a diet that emphasizes on low carbohydrate intake and there are numerous diets from different firms which claim to be effective. These are a couple of the benefits of Atkins diet.

1. EFFECTIVE FOR WEIGHT LOSS

The intake of foods with low carbohydrates is very beneficial in any weight loss program. The Atkins diet usually helps an individual to lose weight without restricting their calorie intake. The end result is a much healthier and fit person.

2. IMPROVES BODY HEALTH

It has been proven that the consumption of the low carbohydrate Atkins diet increases good cholesterol in the body. This is especially important for people with diabetes since it helps in reducing the levels of glucose in the blood.

3. INCORPORATES DIFFERENT TYPES OF FOODS

This is one of the best benefits of Atkins diet that dieters are going to enjoy and thus motivate them to continue dieting. The Atkins diet is inclusive of some very tasty meals that the users can enjoy such as steak. Many people enjoy using the Atkins diet since it provides them freedom in comparison to other restrictive diets.

4. VERY SIMPLE TO USE

Once you have learnt the various carbohydrate counts present in different meals, you can start using the Atkins diet. It is highly advisable that you locate your own position on the provided carbohydrate chart because not every individual has the same qualities. Certain people have increased tolerance for the carbohydrates than others. When using the Atkins diet, you are going to find out your own carbohydrate level as well as how you can use that knowledge to your benefit.

However, people who use the Atkins diet over a long period of time usually suffer from fatigue and frequent migraines. The other disadvantage is rapid weight gain if you stop using this particular diet.

5. MAY NORMALIZE TRIGLYCERIDE AND CHOLESTEROL LEVELS

The Atkins diet is high in fat, specifically saturated fats that many fear contribute to heart problems. However, when saturated fat comes from healthy sources, such as grass-fed beef or coconut oil, it can actually be beneficial for raising HDL cholesterol levels and lowering risk factors for cardiovascular problems. Eating a balanced, unprocessed diet that results in healthy weight loss can also be vital in lowering LDL cholesterol and high triglycerides, which are tied to heart disease and heart attacks.

6. HELPS TREAT POLYCYSTIC OVARIAN SYNDROME (PCOS)

One of the leading risk factors for polycystic ovarian syndrome (PCOS) is having diabetes or being prediabetic, due to the effects of insulin on hormonal balance. PCOS is now the most common endocrine disorder affecting women of reproductive age. It is associated with problems like obesity, hyperinsulinemia, infertility and insulin resistance. While more research is still needed to draw conclusions, some studies have found that a low-carb ketogenic diet leads to significant improvement in PCOS symptoms— including weight, percent of free testosterone, LH/FSH hormone ratio and fasting insulin when followed for a 24-week period.

7. MAY REDUCE DEMENTIA RISK

Low-carb diets have been found to be beneficial for fighting cognitive problems, including dementia, Alzheimer's and narcolepsy. Researchers believe that people with the highest insulin resistance might demonstrate higher levels of inflammation and lower cerebral blood flow (circulation to the brain), therefore less brain plasticity.

THE 4 PHASES OF ATKINS DIET

The Atkins diet has four phases:

Phase 1: Induction

This first phase of the Atkins focuses on dramatic reduction of carbohydrate intake. It's the most restrictive phase of the program; it also results in the fastest weight loss, since your body will begin burning primarily fat for energy when sufficient calories from carbohydrates are not available. This occurs through a process called ketosis, which we'll talk about in more depth later in the course.

Doing Induction successfully requires that you stay on it for at least two weeks, although you can safely do it for months if you have a lot of weight to lose.

If you do not need to lose weight and you want to use this Phase to break addictions to junk food and sugar, you will need to make sure your calorie intake is very high to avoid weight loss. (Women should consume a minimum of 2,000 calories daily; men, 2,800 to 3,000 calories daily)

When you go into Induction you will:

• Limit carbohydrate consumption to 20 grams of Net Carbs (defined below) per day coming primarily from carbohydrates for a minimum of two weeks.

• Satisfy your appetite with foods that combine protein and fat, such as fish, poultry, eggs, lamb, pork and beef; eat limited amounts of hard cheeses (cheeses do contain some carbohydrates) .

• Consume a balance of healthy natural fats such as monounsaturated, polyunsaturated and saturated fats, but avoid manufactured trans fats (e.g. hydrogenated or partially hydrogenated oils).

• Consume carbohydrates in the form of nutrient-dense foods such as leafy green vegetables.

• Drink at least eight glasses of water daily.

Where Have All the Calories Gone?

Here's the first of a many pieces of good news you're going to get as you learn more about the Atkins Diet: You don't need to count calories at this point. You will naturally take in fewer calories because your appetite will be under control with sufficient amounts of protein and fat.

When you give your body too many carbohydrates to metabolize, it burns them for energy. But if you carefully control your carb intake, your body burns fat instead. And that is the secret—if there is one—of the Atkins Diet.

As you read further, you'll see why that's true and how to determine what your net carb intake should be.

What' s a Net Carb?

The Atkins Diet works by restricting carbohydrates, which come from grains, legumes and other plant sources. But most carbohydrates contain fiber, which is not completely digested by the body. Fiber has a great effect on blood sugar, so these substances don't count as carbs on Atkins. So Net Carbs represent the total grams of carbohydrates minus grams of fiber. Net Carbs are the only carbs that you count when you do Atkins.

Successful completion of Induction means transitioning to the next phase: Ongoing Weight Loss.

As good as Induction is for quick, dramatic weight loss, it's important for you to understand that it's only the first Phase. Staying in Phase 1 for too long can become boring. Also, it can lead to a crash-diet mentality where you might assume it's okay to go back to eating anything, because you can always go back and lose the weight all over again by repeating Induction.

You can start with Phase 2 if you don't have a lot of weight to lose, don't want to lose weight at a slower pace, or you find Phase 1 too restrictive.

A person consumes less than 20 grams (g) of carbs each day. At this stage, carbs come mainly from salad and vegetables, which are low in starch.

Phase 2: Ongoing weight loss

When you switch to Ongoing Weight Loss (OWL), your rate of weight loss will naturally slow down. The first week on OWL, you will increase your daily carb intake from 20 to 25 grams; the following week you move to 30 grams of Net Carbs per day, and so on. You should increase intake on a weekly basis until your weight loss slows to one to two pounds each week.

During OWL you'll find out how many grams of carbs you can eat and still lose weight. This is called your personal carb balance.

When you go into OWL you can start adding back nutrient-dense foods like more non-starchy veggies (e.g., asparagus, broccoli); berries like raspberries and strawberries; nuts and seeds like hazelnuts and almonds; and soft cheeses (e.g., cottage cheese).

Phase 2 lasts until you're within 5 to 10 pounds of your weight goal. Successful completion of OWL includes transitioning to the third Phase of the program: Pre-Maintenance.

People gradually introduce nutrient-dense and fiber-rich foods as additional sources of carbs. These foods include nuts, seeds, low carb vegetables, and small amounts of berries. People can also add soft cheeses in this phase.

In phase 2, a person adds:

• 20–25 g of carbs per day during the first week

• 30 g of carbs during the second week

• 30 g each week until weight loss slows to 1–2 pounds a week

The aim of phase 2 is to find out how many carbs an individual can eat while continuing to lose weight. This phase continues until the individual is within 5–10 pounds of their target weight.

Phase 3: Premaintenance

When you're within 5 or 10 pounds of your target weight, it's time to move to Pre-Maintenance.

Now that your weight goal is in sight, the best strategy is to lose the last few pounds very slowly to start a permanently changed way of eating. This Phase lasts until you hit your target weight and maintain it for a month.

Each week in Pre-Maintenance you can add 10 more grams of Net Carbs to your daily allotment. As long as weight loss continues, you can gradually introduce foods such as lentils and other legumes, fruits other than berries, starchy vegetables and whole grains.

When you hit your goal weight and maintain it for at least a month, you've found your carb tolerance level. This is the level of carbohydrate intake at which you will neither gain nor lose weight, and is the key to the final phase, Lifetime Maintenance.

Dieters increase their carbs intake by 10 g each week. Weight loss will now be slow. They can start introducing legumes, such as lentils and beans, fruit, starchy vegetables, and whole grains to the diet.

People continue in this phase until they reach their target weight and maintain it for a month.

Phase 4: Lifetime maintenance

Once you've maintained your goal weight for a month, you've reached Lifetime Maintenance. Lifetime Maintenance is key to the Atkins Diet. In this Phase, the average number of daily grams of Net Carbs ranges from 40 to 120 per day, depending on your metabolism, age, gender, activity level and other factors. If you exercise regularly, you'll probably have a higher carb tolerance level.

In this stage, you will look great and feel great about your progress. But it's important for you to understand that losing weight is only a piece of the puzzle. Atkins isn't just about losing weight; it's also about maintaining health for life. Lifetime

Maintenance is designed to help you to stay healthy throughout your life.

The dieter starts adding a wider range of carbs sources, while carefully monitoring their weight to ensure it does not go up.

Net carb intake will vary between individuals, but it will usually be between 40–120 g a day.

However, these phases are a bit complicated and may not be necessary. You should be able to lose weight and keep it off as long as you stick to the meal plan below.

Some people choose to skip the induction phase altogether and include plenty of vegetables and fruit from the start. This approach can be very effective as well.

Others prefer to just stay in the induction phase indefinitely. This is also known as a very low-carb ketogenic diet (keto).

FOODS TO EAT AND TO BE AVOIDED

On Atkins you can continue to enjoy tasty foods with proteins, fats and fibre, so you'll feel satisfied and full. By eating foods that don't spike your insulin levels, your blood sugar is stabilised so you'll also experience more energy, your cravings disappear and you will feel less bloated.

From day one your eating plan will include green leafy vegetables alongside moderate protein sources such as chicken breast, steak or salmon. These are combined with healthy fats such as avocado, oils, butter, olives and cheese.

For vegetarians, Atkins is still a great way to follow a lower carb, balanced diet. Instead of getting your protein from meat, you can get it from kidney beans, black beans and chickpeas. Plus, you can try incorporating tofu, tempeh, eggs and cheese into your dishes. Fat sources include avocado, oils, butter and olives.

FOODS TO AVOID

You should avoid these foods on the Atkins diet:

- Sugar: Soft drinks, fruit juices, cakes, candy, ice cream, etc.
- Grains: Wheat, spelt, rye, barley, rice.
- Vegetable oils: Soybean oil, corn oil, cottonseed oil, canola oil and a few others.
- Trans fats: Usually found in processed foods with the word "hydrogenated" on the ingredients list.
- "Diet" and "low-fat" foods: These are usually very high in sugar.
- High-carb vegetables: Carrots, turnips, etc (induction only).
- High-carb fruits: Bananas, apples, oranges, pears, grapes (induction only).
- Starches: Potatoes, sweet potatoes (induction only).
- Legumes: Lentils, beans, chickpeas, etc. (induction only).

FOODS TO EAT

You should base your diet around these healthy foods.

• Meats: Beef, pork, lamb, chicken, bacon and others.

• Fatty fish and seafood: Salmon, trout, sardines, etc.

• Eggs: The healthiest eggs are omega-3 enriched or pastured.

• Low-carb vegetables: Kale, spinach, broccoli, asparagus and others.

• Full-fat dairy: Butter, cheese, cream, full-fat yogurt.

• Nuts and seeds: Almonds, macadamia nuts, walnuts, sunflower seeds, etc.

• Healthy fats: Extra virgin olive oil, coconut oil, avocados and avocado oil.

As long as you base your meals around a fatty protein source with vegetables or nuts and some healthy fats, you will lose weight. It's that simple.

BEVERAGES

Here there are some drinks that are acceptable on the Atkins diet.

• Water: As always, water should be your go-to beverage.

• Coffee: Many studies show that coffee is high in antioxidants and quite healthy.

• Green tea: A very healthy beverage.

Alcohol is also fine in small amounts. Stick to dry wines with no added sugars and avoid high-carb drinks like beer.

CAN BE EATEN

There are many delicious foods you can eat on the Atkins diet.

This includes foods like bacon, heavy cream, cheese and dark chocolate.

Many of these are generally considered fattening because of the high fat and calorie content.

However, when you're on a low-carb diet, your body increases its use of fat as an energy source and suppresses your appetite, reducing the risk of overeating and weight gain.

HEALTHY LOW-CARB SNACKS

Most people feel that their appetite goes down on the Atkins diet.

They tend to feel more than satisfied with 3 meals per day (sometimes only 2).

However, if you feel hungry between meals, here are a few quick healthy snacks:

• Leftovers.

• A hard-boiled egg or two.

• A piece of cheese.

• A piece of meat.

• A handful of nuts.

• Some Greek yogurt.

• Berries and whipped cream.

• Baby carrots (careful during induction).

• Fruits (after induction).

ATKINS MENU FOR ONE WEEK

This is a sample menu for one week on the Atkins diet.

It's suitable for the induction phase, but you should add more higher-carb vegetables and some fruits as you move on to the other phases.

Monday

• Breakfast: Eggs and vegetables, fried in coconut oil.

• Lunch: Chicken salad with olive oil, and a handful of nuts.

• Dinner: Steak and veggies.

Tuesday

• Breakfast: Bacon and eggs.

• Lunch: Leftover chicken and veggies from the night before.

• Dinner: Bunless cheeseburger, with vegetables and butter.

Wednesday

• Breakfast: Omelet with veggies, fried in butter.

• Lunch: Shrimp salad with some olive oil.

• Dinner: Ground-beef stir fry, with veggies.

Thursday

• Breakfast: Eggs and veggies, fried in coconut oil.

• Lunch: Leftover stir fry from dinner the night before.

• Dinner: Salmon with butter and vegetables.

Friday

• Breakfast: Bacon and eggs.

• Lunch: Chicken salad with olive oil and a handful of nuts.

• Dinner: Meatballs with vegetables.

Saturday

• Breakfast: Omelet with various vegetables, fried in butter.

• Lunch: Leftover meatballs from the night before.

• Dinner: Pork chops with vegetables.

Sunday

• Breakfast: Bacon and eggs.

• Lunch: Leftover pork chops from the night before.

• Dinner: Grilled chicken wings, with some salsa and veggies.

Make sure to include a variety of different vegetables in your diet.

A simple Shopping List for the Atkins Diet. It's a good rule to shop at the perimeter of the store. This is usually where the whole foods are found.

Eating organic is not necessary, but always go for the least processed option that fits your budget.

• Meats: Beef, chicken, lamb, pork, bacon.

• Fatty fish: Salmon, trout, etc.

• Shrimp and shellfish.

• Eggs.

• Dairy: Greek yogurt, heavy cream, butter, cheese.

• Vegetables: Spinach, kale, lettuce, tomatoes, broccoli, cauliflower, asparagus, onions, etc.

• Berries: Blueberries, strawberries, etc.

• Nuts: Almonds, macadamia nuts, walnuts, hazelnuts, etc.

• Seeds: Sunflower seeds, pumpkin seeds, etc.

• Fruits: Apples, pears, oranges.

• Coconut oil.

• Olives.

• Extra virgin olive oil.

- Dark chocolate.

- Avocados.

- Condiments: Sea salt, pepper, turmeric, cinnamon, garlic, parsley, etc.

It's highly recommended to clear your pantry of all unhealthy foods and ingredients. This includes ice cream, sodas, breakfast cereals, breads, juices and baking ingredients like sugar and wheat flour.

THE 11 DIET SWAPS THAT MAKE THE LOW-CARB DIET EASY

Replace pasta with spiralised vegetables

Try making your own alternative to pasta at home by spiralizing courgette, carrot or other veg. You can buy a gadget to help you make perfect swirls or just use a grater. Serve with chicken or fish and make your own spicy tomato sauce or a tasty creamy sauce.

Get a chocolate hit that's low-carb

Swap your afternoon chocolate bar for an Atkins bar, which contains a fraction of the carbs yet tastes just as great (or even better!). A filling 60g Atkins bar contains 1-3g carbs, compared to 30-40g in a typical chocolate bar.

Control your coffee choice

Avoid high sugar milk from your local coffee shop and make your own version using unsweetened soya milk, espresso and a dollop of sugar-free whipped cream on top. A tall latte is typically around 17 grams sugar, compared to two grams for your home-made version!

Stick to wine

Alcohol can be loaded with carbs so avoid beer, cider and sugary cocktails and stick to wine. It's your choice whether you prefer red or white, but pinot noir is typically lower in carbs than other reds. For white, stick to crisp, dry wines for fewer carbs. Remember to drink water between each drink; not only it will stop you from getting a hangover but you'll feel fuller and less likely to give into cravings.

Do your own barbecue meat

Having a BBQ? Don't buy store-bought meats, which come with cereal fillers, or sugary marinades. Save pounds and lbs, by making your own BBQ feast. Skewer chicken pieces with vegetables, for healthy, colourful kebabs, or make your own burgers using mince meat, spices and a bit of chopped chilli and avoid the heavy burgers you find in shops.

Go no carb Mexican

Most Mexican food is great on Atkins with plenty of protein, guacamole, salsas and salads but use large lettuce leaves to wrap up the tasty fillings rather than carb-heavy tortillas.

Have a fry up without the carbs

By all, means enjoy a full English breakfast, but omit the carb heavy beans, hash browns and toast – and double up on bacon, eggs and mushrooms (the best bits!)

Cauliflower pizza is actually really nice

Might sound a little odd, but you'd never know you were eating cauliflower, and it's so easy to make. Just cut some cauliflower into florets, blend into small pieces, then mix with mozzarella, parmesan, seasoning, garlic and 2 eggs. Spread into a pizza shape on a baking sheet covered with baking powder, bake for 20 mins, then add the desired toppings and bake for a further 10 minutes.

Make the salad the main event

Salads can be great but can also be boring…don't just stick to limp lettuce, make yours a tasty treat by adding olives, feta, sliced avocado, sliced jalapenos, chorizo slices, crushed nuts and other low carb additions.

Don't get too hungry

Many people skimp on calories when trying to lose weight and it just doesn't work. On Atkins, we recommend three meals with two between-meal snacks. So your blood sugar levels stabilise and you never feel hungry. Try one of our tasty bars for one of your snacks for a mid-morning or afternoon treat.

Try an Atkins Bar

Atkins bars are a great way to snack between meals and not ruin your eating plan. They're low in sugar as well as carbs so are ideal for if you're out about on the go or need a pick me up pre- or post workout.

How to Follow the Atkins Diet when eating out

It's actually very easy to follow the Atkins diet at most restaurants.

1. Get extra vegetables instead of bread, potatoes or rice.

2. Order a meal based on fatty meat or fatty fish.

3. Get some extra sauce, butter or olive oil with your meal.

HOW THE ATKINS DIET IS BETTER THAN OTHER POPULAR DIETS

Atkins diet marginally better than rivals, Atkins and keto are two of the best-known low-carb diets.

Both stipulate a drastic reduction in high-carb foods, including sweets, sugary drinks, breads, grains, fruits, legumes, and potatoes.

Though these diets are similar, they have differences as well. The Atkins diet is one of the best-known diets worldwide. It's a low-carb, moderate-protein, high-fat diet.

Though Atkins has evolved to offer a variety of plans, the original version (now called Atkins 20) is still the most popular.

The keto diet

The keto, or ketogenic, diet is a very-low-carb, moderate-protein, high-fat diet plan.

It was first used to treat children who experienced seizures, but researchers discovered that it may benefit other people as well.

The goal of the keto diet is to get your body into the metabolic state of ketosis, during which it uses fat rather than sugar from carbs as its main energy source.

In ketosis, your body runs on ketones, which are compounds that are formed upon the breakdown of the fat in your food or the fat stored in your body.

To achieve and maintain ketosis, most people need to limit their total carb intake to 20–50 grams per day. Macronutrient ranges for the keto diet are typically under 5% of calories from carbs, 10-30% from protein, and 65-90% from fat.

Similarities and differences

Keto and Atkins share certain similarities but also differ greatly in some respects.

- Similarities

As they're both low-carb diets, Atkins and keto are alike in some ways.

In fact, Phase 1 (Induction) of the Atkins diet is similar to the keto diet, as it restricts net carbs to 25 grams per day. In doing so, your body likely enters ketosis and starts burning fat as its main source of fuel.

What's more, both diets may result in weight loss by decreasing the number of calories you eat. Many carbs — particularly refined carbs like sweets, chips, and sugary drinks — are high in calories and may contribute to weight gain.

Both Atkins and keto require you to eliminate these high-calorie, carb-rich foods, which makes it easier to cut calories and lose weight.

- Differences

Atkins and keto have certain differences as well.

While keto is a moderate-protein approach, with about 20% of calories coming from protein, the Atkins diet allows for up to 30% of calories from protein, depending on the phase.

Additionally, on the keto diet, you want to keep your body in ketosis by extremely limiting your carb intake.

On the other hand, the Atkins diet has you gradually increase your carb intake, which will eventually kick your body out of ketosis.

Due to this flexible carb limit, Atkins allows for a wider variety of foods, such as more fruits and vegetables and even some grains.

Overall, Atkins is a less restrictive approach, as you don't have to monitor ketones or stick to certain macronutrient targets to stay in ketosis.

Potential benefits

Though once considered unhealthy, low-carb diets have now been shown to offer various health benefits.

- Weight loss

Low-carb diets may result in more weight loss than other diet plans.

In a review of six popular diets, including Atkins, the Zone diet, the Ornish diet, and Jenny Craig, Atkins resulted in the most weight loss after six months .

A similar study found that Atkins was the most likely among 7 popular diets to result in meaningful weight loss 6–12 months after starting the plan.

Though more restrictive than Atkins, the keto diet may aid weight loss as well. Research indicates that being in ketosis decreases appetite, thereby removing one of the biggest barriers to weight loss — constant hunger.

Ketogenic diets also preserve your muscle mass, meaning that most of the lost weight is more likely to be a result of fat loss.

In one 12-month study, participants on a low-calorie keto diet lost about 44 pounds (20 kg) with few losses in muscle mass, compared to the standard low-calorie group, which only lost 15 pounds (7 kg).

Additionally, ketogenic diets maintain your resting metabolic rate (RMR), or the number of calories you burn at rest, whereas other low-calorie diets may cause your RMR to decrease.

- Blood sugar control

Research indicates that low-carb diets can benefit blood sugar control.

In fact, the American Diabetes Association recently revised the Standards of Medical Care, a document outlining how healthcare providers should manage and treat diabetes, to include low-carb diets as a safe and effective option for people with type 2 diabetes.

Low-carb diets have been shown to decrease the need for diabetes medications and improve levels of hemoglobin A1c (HgbA1c), a marker of long-term blood sugar control.

One 24-week study in 14 obese adults with type 2 diabetes on the Atkins diet found that in addition to losing weight, participants lowered their HgbA1c levels and decreased their need for diabetes medications.

Another 12-month study in 34 overweight adults noted that participants on a keto diet had lower HgbA1c levels, experienced more weight loss, and were more likely to discontinue diabetes medications than those on a moderate-carb, low-fat diet.

Other benefits

Research suggests that low-carb, higher-fat diets may improve certain heart disease risk factors.

Low-carb diets may reduce triglyceride levels and increase HDL (good) cholesterol, thereby decreasing the ratio of triglycerides to HDL cholesterol.

A high triglyceride-to-HDL ratio is an indicator of poor heart health and has been linked to increased heart disease risk.

A review including over 1,300 people found that those on the Atkins diet had greater decreases in triglycerides and more significant increases in HDL cholesterol than individuals following a low-fat diet.

Low-carb diets have also been associated with other benefits, including improved mental health and digestion.

WHAT YOU SHOULD KNOW BEFORE YOU BEGIN ATKINS DIET

Things You Should Know Before Starting the Atkins Diet

1. Atkins was the staple diet of the early 2000s.

Though Atkins began in 1972 when Robert C. Atkins released his book, Dr. Atkins' Diet Revolution, it didn't become crazy popular until the early 2000s, when he released his second book.

2. Krispy Kreme and the pasta industry were not fans.

The doughnut giant blamed Atkins and other low-carb diets like it for a huge drop in sales.

3. The key is to eat low carb, not low cal.

Atkins works by reducing sugar and carbs (which later turn into sugar) so that the body doesn't burn these for fuel but burns fat instead. In that sense, you're counting your net carb intake—AKA, those bites of bread and pasta you just can't resist—rather than count calories.

4. There's two diet plans to suit your needs.

If you follow Atkins, there are 2 plans to choose from: Atkins 20 and Atkins 40. With Atkins 20, you start by eating only 20 net carbs per day and eventually add more carbs (and food options) as you move through its four phases. This plan is recommended for people who have 40 or more pounds to lose.

With Atkins 40 you can eat, you guessed it, 40 net carbs per day. With this plan you eat three meals and two snacks per day, and you have way more food options. This option is good for people who have less than 40 pounds to lose, are breast feeding, or just need a little more variety in their meals.

5. Atkins lets you eat lots and lots of cheese.

A diet that lets you eat cheese? Yup, it exists. Atkins advocates eating both dairy and healthy fats, so you can keep munching on that fancy brie, or have yourself a little pat of butter—no problem (as long as you account for the net carbs, of course).

6. You'll have to pack on the protein.

Atkins is big on protein with every meal. In fact, at three 4- to 6-ounce servings on Atkins 40, it's a large part of your daily food intake. The good news is you can get your protein from lots of foods, including eggs, poultry, seafood, buffalo (hmmm), and even bacon.

7. You'll also have to put your alcohol behind lock and key.

Unfortunately, alcohol is not a part of either Atkins 20 or 40. Though the occasional glass of wine is no biggie, alcohol consumption slows down weight loss, so if you're really looking to lose weight, you should avoid drinking a whole bottle. Approved alcohols include: wine, rye, scotch, vodka, and gin—but lose the juice, tonic water, and non-diet soda, they'll add unwanted carbs and ruin your hard work.

8. Vegetarians and vegans can get in on the action too.

Atkins is an EOD (Equal Opportunity Diet) so non-meat eaters can follow the food plan by getting their protein from eggs, cheese, and soy products. Vegans can eat seeds, nuts, soy products, soy and rice cheeses, and high-protein grains like quinoa.

9. The diet has been recently corrected to include a lot more plants.

Atkins recently released a hip new version of its diet plan called Eco-Atkins. The new diet focuses on getting 31 percent of calories from plant proteins, 43 percent from plant fats and 26 percent from plant carbs, so basically this is the diet for vegetarians. There's little guidance on the diet (it doesn't even have an online presence), making it kind of hard to follow.

10. They have frozen meals and recipes galore to keep you on track.

Let's be real: Frozen meals are definite not the most appetizing thing in the world, but they do cut out the math of having to calculate net carbs yourself (they're printed on the box), and they're fast. Atkins has a variety of frozen meals, including breakfast options, a range of American options, and even global choices. My recommendation? Try the beef merlot or meatloaf—they're bomb. However, save yourself the disappointment and steer clear of the chicken options.

11. You can also get fresh meals delivered.

Not into frozen, but also not into cooking? That's cool. If you've got the cash, you can get fresh Atkins meals delivered to you. You can subscribe and get a personalized meal plan, or order a la carte.

12. Counting carbs? There's an app for that.

Atkins wouldn't make it in the 21st century if it didn't have a carb-counting app. The app functions like most others of its kind, but in addition to having the nutrition info for basically every grocery item on the planet, it includes data for Atkins products and recipes. So basically, you just type in words and never actually have to do math to figure out your carb intake, making dieting a no-brainer.

13. It's gonna get worse before it gets better.

If you're dieting, it means you're most likely really changing your eating habits, and that's obviously not going to be easy. People on Atkins tend to have initial some effects, including headaches, dizziness, weakness, fatigue and constipation. Of course, these side effects might occur with any diet, so it really is up to you: Is the gain worth the pain?

14. It may or may not have other health benefits.

Atkins marketing never fails to mention that aside from helping to lose weight, the diet plan also reduces risk for heart disease and diabetes.

15. It initially advocated unlimited cheese and meat.

Part of the reason why some doctors were initially skeptical of Atkins is because at first, it advocated eating cheese, meats, and fats liberally. Since then, the diet has undergone some changes, namely advocating for more moderation in dining on meat and dairy. Some experts are still not entirely convinced about a high-fat and protein diet, but little extensive research has been done.

16. Some prolific stars are fans of the diet.

Many stars have been rumored to use Atkins to maintain their weight.

17. It's kind of expensive.

Atkins, by virtue of making you eat fresh, non-processed food, is a pricey diet to maintain.

TIPS ABOUT HOW TO DO ATKINS DIET SUCCESSFULLY

Tips for Success on the Atkins Diet

Following these 16 tips will help you stay on track and get started on Atkins:

1. Understand what you are eating and how Atkins works. Atkins is all about eating right. You'll learn which foods your body needs to lose or maintain weight, how to easily reduce the amount of added sugar and other empty carbs and in your diet, how to understand what that Nutritional Facts label really says and more.

2. Atkins, customized for you. Depending on how much weight you have to lose, Atkins has a plan that will work for you: Atkins 20, the original plan that has you consuming 20 Net Carbs a day or Atkins 40, where you consume 40 grams of Net Carbs a day and a full range of food options.

3. Count your carbs. Understand what Net Carbs are and how to calculate them, using the handy Carb Counter in combination with the Acceptable Foods lists for your plan.

4. Be sensible, not obsessive, about portions. There's no need to count calories on Atkins, but you should use common sense. You probably could guess that too many calories will slow down weight loss, but too few will slow down your metabolism—and, therefore, weight loss. You only need worry about calories if, despite following Atkins to the letter, you cannot lose weight. Depending upon your height, age and metabolism, you may need to play with the following calorie ranges to lose weight: Women, should stick with 1,500–1,800 calories a day and men should stick with 1,800–2,200 calories per day.

5. Eat regularly. That's right, no starving! Regardless of which phase you're in, eat three regular-sized meals plus two snacks every day. Or, if you prefer, have four or five small meals throughout the day.Eating every few hours maintains blood sugar and energy levels and keeps your appetite under control. Eat until you're satisfied but not stuffed. Atkins has a full range of products,

including frozen meals, shakes, bars and treats that make it convenient and easy to stay on track.

6. Include protein in every meal. Make sure you are having 4 to 6 ounces of protein at breakfast, lunch and dinner. Men can have up to 8 ounces. You can choose eggs, meat (lean or fatty is fine), poultry; even marbled cuts of beef are fine. When leaner cuts are used, be sure to ensure enough of olive oil or other healthy oils on salads and cooked veggies.

7. Savor foods with natural fats. Fat makes food taste good and is filling so you eat less. In fact, dietary fat is key to the Atkins program, and to overall good health. All fats except manufactured trans fats (hydrogenated or partially hydrogenated oils) are a healthy part of Atkins.

8. Steer clear of added sugar. Added sugar comes in many forms and is found in most soft drinks and countless other foods. All are high in carbs and calories and empty of other nutrients. Instead, sweeten beverages with non-caloric sweeteners (stevia, sucralose—marketed as Splenda™—saccharin or xylitol.) Count each packet as 1

gram of Net Carbs and don't exceed three a day.

9. Eat veggies. Be sure to consume at least 12 to 15 grams of carbohydrates in the form of Foundation Vegetables each day. From the start, you'll meet the USDA's recommended intake of at least five daily servings of vegetables. You'll also be getting plenty of fiber, which plays a key role in blood sugar management, and, of course, regularity. Fiber also helps you feel full, and helps with weight control.

10. Enjoy eating—at home, in a restaurant, wherever. Unlike other diets that instill a fear of eating or require the purchase of expensive, pre-packaged meals, Atkins is all about eating delicious whole foods. You'll learn how to choose the right foods whether you're dining in or out, whether you're at a fast-food place or an ethnic restaurant, on the road for business or on vacation. Soon you'll know how to make the right choices and stay on track.

11. Drink up. Water and other fluids like tea and coffee (in moderation) encourage your body to let go of water weight—plus water

is just plain healthy. Aim for eight 8-ounce glasses each day.

12. Take daily supplements. In combination with a whole-foods diet, supplements are a good protocol on any weight loss program. Take a daily multivitamin with minerals, including potassium, magnesium and calcium, but without iron—unless you are iron deficient. Also omega-3s in the form of fish oil or an alternative is a good therapeutic tool.

13. Get moving. There are countless benefits to physical activity and exercise as a natural partner to a healthy diet. Brisk walking, swimming and other fun activities are an integral component of Atkins. And the more muscle you build, the more calories you'll burn. You may want to wait a couple of weeks after starting Atkins to begin a new fitness regimen—or ramp up your existing one. And if you have a lot of weight to lose, you may want to start slowly with short walks or water aerobics.

14. Track your successes. We're talking about both pounds and health indicators. Weigh and measure yourself at the chest, waist and hips once a week. Also, keep a

journal of food and fluid intake, as well as challenges and victories. Numerous studies indicate journal keepers are more successful at weight management than others. Get some baseline tests before you start Atkins—and 3 to 6 months later for follow up lipid levels. Prepare to be amazed at how much healthier they've become.

15. Get support from friends and family. Let the important people in your life know how they're doing and feeling. An Atkins buddy can share the ups and downs of their journey. Also, be sure to join the Community Forum at Atkins.com.

16. Plan ahead. Stock your kitchen with the right food and snacks. Decide on your meals before you go grocery shopping so you don't fall back on your old (high-carb) food choices.

The Wrong Way to Do Atkins

1. Misconception: Atkins can be used as a short-term or crash diet.

Reality: If you do Induction for two weeks to drop 10 pounds and then go back to your old way of eating, you will be treating it as a crash diet. But that goes against everything I recommend, and will lead to problems in the long run.

2. Misconception: You can lose weight doing Atkins, then return to your old way of eating.

Reality: Do this, and as with your past attempts, you will neglect to change those eating habits that ensure you always regain lost weight.

3. Misconception: You can focus only on losing weight and minimize the maintenance aspects.

Reality: Any weight loss program that does not flow into weight maintenance is doomed to failure. The eating plan you will follow during Lifetime Maintenance is likely to be something between your menu during the Induction phase and the way you ate before you started Atkins.

4. Misconception: You can eat any food so long you do not exceed 20 grams of carbs a day.

Reality: If you eat junk foods or other nutrient deficient carbohydrate foods instead of vegetables and other nutrient-dense foods, you will miss most of the benefits I write about and you certainly will not be fostering long-term health.

5. Misconception: You can use Atkins for weight loss, but you don't have to bother with exercise and supplements if you don't have any health problems.

Reality: If you don't supplement with vitanutrients and exercise regularly, you may take off pounds, but you will miss out on important health benefits. And everyone needs exercise: It is not related only to weight loss.

6. Misconception: You can just continue to do Induction until you lose all of your weight.

Reality: You will lose weight more quickly if you continue doing Induction, but you won't learn how to keep that weight off permanently if you don't move through the four phases. More important, you will miss out on the benefits of the phytochemicals present in health-promoting carbohydrate foods.

7. Misconception: You can go back to eating your favorite foods after you lose weight. Reality: Your favorite foods may well be your problem foods. Unless you acknowledge and learn how to deal with your addictions, you are doomed to regain your weight and fall back into the dangerous cycle of high blood sugar and overproduction of insulin.

8. Misconception: You can do Induction during the week and binge on weekends and still lose or maintain weight.

Reality: When you do Atkins during the week and then cheat on the weekends, for several days after your binge, you are no longer burning fat. At most, you could be in the fat-burning state for only three days each week. In addition, you may have overstimulated your insulin response, increasing the metabolic risk factors underlying your weight problem. Remember that when you burn fat, dietary fat is also being burned. However, if you combine high carbs with high fat-the typical American diet-you can be increasing your cardiovascular risks.

9. Misconception: You can do Atkins while following a low-fat regimen.

Reality: To encourage your body to burn its own stores of fat, you need to reduce the amount of carbohydrates you eat, meaning you need to eat primarily foods rich in protein and fat. Remember that essential fatty acids play a role in normal metabolic function. Fat also plays a role in stabilizing blood sugar and increasing satiety. If fat intake is too low, you will not burn fat aggresively. Moreover, excess protein converts to glucose and can keep fat from becoming the primary fuel.

8 WEEKS ATKINS DIET MEAL PLAN FOOD YOU CAN ENJOY AND RECIPES FOR EACH PHASE

Anyone who is committed to doing Atkins properly needs to follow these rules to the letter. Remember that it takes two to three days for the body to switch to fat burning. One cheat and you're back to a glucose-burning metabolism. You can lose the effects of two or three days of fat burning with one cheat. So if you have the misguided belief that you can do Atkins all week and then indulge over the weekend, don't expect to see dramatic results.

Now to the meal plans. Follow this menu for the first week, then repeat it for the second week.

Meal Plans for the Atkins Diet

The types of meals that you should be eating will vary depending upon which stage of the diet you are at: Induction, Ongoing Weight-loss, Pre-maintenance or Maintenance.

Menu for the Induction Stage

Breakfast:

• Ham or bacon with eggs (fried or scrambled) and, to drink, decaffeinated tea or coffee.

Lunch:

• Bacon cheeseburger (making sure you serve it without the bun to avoid the carbohydrates) accompanied by a small salad and a glass of water.

Dinner:

• Prawn cocktail as a starter – the sauce should be made from mustard and mayonnaise.

• Clear consommé – this is a specialised kind of light soup made mainly from a kind of refined stock. This can be quite tricky to make so, unless you are particularly handy in the kitchen, you may prefer to search your local supermarket for a good, low carbohydrate brand Meat (choose any from the following: a steak, chops, a portion of fish, fowl or a roast) to be served with a salad.

• Sugar free jelly accompanied by a small serving of whipped cream (make sure this is also sugar free) for dessert.

Menu for the Ongoing Weight-loss Stage

Breakfast:

• Cheese omelette to be accompanied by some bran based crisp bread (to an amount containing carbohydrate to the value of 2 grams).

• To drink - decaffeinated tea or coffee and also 3 ounces of tomato juice

Lunch:

• A chicken, cheese, ham and egg salad. For the dressing keep it simple with an oil and vinegar based dressing.

• Herbal iced tea.

Dinner:

• A seafood salad.

• Poached salmon with a small portion of vegetables (avoid root vegetables to minimise your carbohydrate intake).

• A small portion of strawberries for dessert with double cream (unsweetened).

Menu for the Pre-maintenance and Maintenance Stages

Breakfast:

• Cheese and spinach omelette

• Half of one cantaloupe

• Bran based crisp bread with butter (to an amount containing carbohydrate to the value of 4 grams)

• Decaffeinated tea or coffee to drink

Lunch:

• Roast chicken accompanied by a small portion of vegetables and a salad. Try a green salad with a creamy garlic dressing

• Soda water to drink

Dinner:

• French onion soup to start

• Salad with onions, tomatoes and carrots with a dressing (without carbohydrate in it)

• Veal chops (these can be breaded, but not too heavily as this will contain carbohydrates) accompanied by a small portion of vegetables and half of a jacket potato topped with sour cream and chives

• A small portion of fresh fruit dessert compote

• 1 glass of dry wine (or, if you prefer, two white wine spritzers – this is the old fashioned kind with soda water rather than the modern version of the spritzer served with lemonade)

More Simple Meal Ideas with Atkins

There are plenty of meals which can complement your Atkins diet. Below are some ideas to get you started.

- Bacon, celery, walnut and avocado salad

- Thai coconut curry

- Chilli and pepper marinated steak

- Chicken kebabs with peanut dipping sauce

- Beef and mushroom skewers

- Pork in a creamy paprika sauce

- Stuffed, baked chicken wrapped in parma ham

- Baked marrow stuffed with cheeses

- Haddock stuffed with leek and spinach sauce

- Tandoori chicken skewers

- Lemon seafood salad

- Large mushrooms stuffed with goats cheese

- Eggs Benedict accompanied by hollandaise sauce

- Pork with a stilton based sauce to accompany

- Vegetable curry

ONE-WEEK INDUCTION MENU

Monday

BREAKFAST

- Two scrambled eggs
- Two turkey sausages

LUNCH

- Greek salad made with Romaine lettuce, half a tomato, feta cheese, olives and dill vinaigrette Small can of tuna

DINNER

- Veal Scallops with White Wine Caper Sauce*
- Sauteed spinach Gelatin dessert made with sucralose topped with whipped cream

SNACK

- Controlled carb strawberry shake

Tuesday

BREAKFAST
- Crustless Quiche*
- Two tomato slices

LUNCH
- Chicken salad served over chopped cucumber, radishes and watercress

DINNER
- Maple Mustard-Glazed Salmon*
- Sauteed broccoli with red pepper
- Small green salad with vinaigrette

SNACK
- Ten to twenty olives

Wednesday

BREAKFAST
- Smoked salmon and cream cheese roll-ups Two hard-boiled eggs

LUNCH
- Homemade Chicken Soup*

DINNER
- Broiled steak Oven-Fried Turnips*
- Arugula and Boston lettuce salad

SNACK
- Turkey,   Romaine   lettuce, mayonnaise roll-up

Thursday

BREAKFAST
- Western omelette with green salsa

LUNCH
- Vegetable broth with shredded white radish Shrimp salad over greens

DINNER
- Turkey   Cutlets   with   Green Peppercorn Sauce*   Cauliflower-Leek Puree*
- Gelatin dessert made with sucralose topped with whipped cream

SNACK
- One ounce Swiss cheese

Friday

BREAKFAST
- Two ounces cream cheese sprinkled with cinnamon and flax seeds
- Two Bran-a-Crisp crackers

LUNCH
- Chef's salad with blue cheese dressing

DINNER
- Pork burgers Creamy Red Cabbage Slaw*
- Broiled portobello mushrooms with sesame oil

SNACK
- Mocha granita

Saturday

BREAKFAST
- Whitefish salad
- Two tomato slices

LUNCH
- Ham, spinach and cheese omelette
- Mixed green salad

DINNER
- Herbed-Roast Chicken with Lemon*
- Buttered green beans
- Italian Almond Cream*

SNACK
- Celery stuffed with Roasted Garlic and Vegetable Dip*

Sunday

BREAKFAST
- One and a half slices Zucchini Nut Bread* Two ounces cream cheese

LUNCH
- Broiled cheeseburger
- Large mixed green salad with two tomato slices

DINNER
- Cajun Pork Chops*
- Sauteed kale with garlic

SNACK
- Controlled carb vanilla shake

HOW THE ATKINS SYSTEM OF EATING CAN BE ADAPTED TO YOUR INDIVIDUALS NEEDS, EVEN PROVIDING YOU WITH TASTY DIABETIC-FRIENDLY RECIPES

For many, cutting out and minimising carbohydrate intake can be very difficult. There are many ways that you can try and make this a little easier however.

• The Atkins' diet has many tips on how to avoid carbohydrates and also additional helpful substitutes.

• You can order substitute products from the Atkins diet, such as Atkins bake mix, which reduce the carbohydrate content of your meals.

• The above reduced-carbohydrate bake mix minimises the carbohydrate content of all your baking so you can have cakes, breads, etc.

• Use sugar substitutes instead of regular sugar which should have less 'food energy'. Be sure to check the packets though to make sure this is the case – some substitutes are better than others.

• Search your local stores for controlled-carbohydrate pasta so that you can still enjoy your favourite Italian dishes from time to time.

• Use reduced-carbohydrate bread instead of regular brands. By doing this you can still enjoy a sandwich or two while you are on your diet.

• Sometimes this high-protein diet can become quite monotonous if you do not know how to vary your meals. Experiment with different ways of cooking things – use different spices and seasonings to add variety and interest to potentially similar meals. However be careful that you take note of the ingredients that you use when making your sauces. Ingredients such as refined white flour, honey and sugar can impede your weight loss when following the Atkins diet.

If you are finding it difficult to lose weight, or would like to lose more, then the above areas might provide you with some indication as to either where you are going wrong or where there are areas that you can reduce your carbohydrate intake even more.

ATKINS DIET FOR VEGETARIANS

The Atkins diet is much harder for vegetarians because meat proteins are an integral part of the diet and the suggested meal plans. It is likely that vegetarians will have much less successful results than those who eat meat, and involve more planning and care, so you may wish to look into alternative diet plans. If you are positive that you wish to go on the Atkins diet you should consult with your doctor or nutritionist first. It is likely that your meal plans will feature eggs and cheese heavily in order for you to consume sufficient amounts of protein.

THE ATKINS DIET AND VEGANS

The advice for vegetarians as above is relevant here, however it is likely that vegans will have to look for an alternative diet as you obviously will not have the protein sources listed above as options.

Vegan diets contain too much carbohydrate and it is extremely unlikely that you would be able to make a success of your Atkins diet in combination with this.

IDEAS TO FACILITATE YOUR VEGETARIAN ATKINS DIET

The following tips should help you to get you started on your vegetarian version of the Atkins diet.

• Research the traditional Atkins diet in detail. Make a note of any potential areas you will need to be aware of, for example keeping your protein levels up by increasing the quantity of cheese, tofu and egg you consume to make up for the fact you are not eating meat.

• Ensure that you check the labels of what you eat to minimise the amount of carbohydrates you consume, particularly in the first weeks of your Atkins diet when carbohydrate consumption should be as low as possible. The carbohydrates you do eat should come from berries, seeds, fresh vegetables and small amounts of fruit and nuts. Processed foods, sugar and white flour should all be removed from your diet. Remember that, while you do need to keep your protein intake up, foods such as cheese and tofu do contain some carbohydrate so you should take this into consideration when calculating your carbohydrate consumption.

• The fact that your sources of protein already up your carbohydrate intake means that you will have to be even more careful than meat eaters of the vegetables and fruits, etc. that you eat to ensure you are consuming those with the lowest carbohydrates in. This will allow you to try and even out and make up for the carbohydrates contained in your protein sources.

• After you have restricted your carbohydrate intake as much as possible, during the later stages of the diet, you can then very slowly reintroduce foods which have a higher carbohydrate concentration such as oats, cous cous, barley and vegetables with over 10 per cent carbohydrates in, most root vegetables for example.

• If you are comfortable including fish in your diet then this is a useful way of complementing your Atkins diet. This will add variety to your meals and also reduce the intake of carbohydrates instead which will hinder you sticking to the diet properly and, in doing so, also hinder your weight loss.

The stricter your vegetarian diet is, the harder it will be to stick to the Atkins diet. Protein is a very large part of the Atkins diet and so avoiding meat, and even fish, limits your options greatly.

Anyone should consult a health professional, nutritionist or medical practitioner before embarking upon any new nutrition plan or a drastic change in diet. If however you are a vegetarian this is even more applicable advice to ensure that you get the best out of your new diet plan whilst still getting the necessary nutrients.

ATKINS DIET SIDE EFFECTS

Typical side effects usually experienced by following the Atkins Diet.

There are many side effects that people tend to experience while following the Atkins diet. Some are just a short term inconvenience; however, some experts believe that the Atkins diet can also have a more long term detrimental effect on your health.

Short Term and Instant Side Effects of Atkins

There are various side effects which people can experience while following the Atkins diet. Different people experience different variations and combinations of the below symptoms shortly after beginning the Atkins diet:

• Fatigue

• Dizziness and generally feeling weak

• Insomnia

• Nausea

• Halitosis

• Constipation

Causes of These Short Term Side Effects

Any sudden, drastic change in diet can cause your body to react and in doing so cause different side effects. These may be very different for different people, however it is likely that you will experience at least a couple of the above symptoms. The symptoms of fatigue and feeling weak are a result of your body altering the energy source it uses. With the decrease in carbohydrate intake (its preferred energy source) your body must find other energy sources to use which can often make you feel lethargic, weak and sluggish. As you and your body get used to this change you will not experience these symptoms as much.

LONG TERM SIDE EFFECTS OF ATKINS

Much research has been done into whether the Atkins diet has more serious long-term side effects. While much of this research is inconclusive, many believe that the Atkins diet can have quite a detrimental effect upon your health, particularly if followed over a long period of time. Many believe that the likelihood of having or experiencing the following is much increased by being on the Atkins diet for any length of time:

• Heart disease

- Cancer

- Osteoporosis

- Premature aging

- Cataracts

- Kidney problems

- Weak bones

CAUSES OF THESE LONG TERM SIDE EFFECTS

These side effects are generally agreed to be as a result of the Atkins diet's reliance on what is essentially quite an imbalanced diet. The fact that many key nutrients do not feature in the diet is a cause of concern for many experts. Dr. Atkins emphasises the importance of taking vitamins and other supplements to make up for this. However most nutritionists agree that taking pills to get these nutrients is no substitute for consuming the correct foods to get them naturally. The importance of dairy in your diet cannot be underestimated for the benefits it provides your body, specifically in ensuring your bones are strong and healthy.

How to Minimise these Side Effects

The best way to minimise these side effects is to do as much research as possible in advance. Similarly you should consult at length with your medical practitioner and a dietician or nutritionist. By learning all of the facts and risks then you can embark upon your diet as healthily as possible and taking as many precautions as possible.

ATKINS & ATHLETES

Athletes require a great deal of energy in order to perform to their optimum level. The best energy source for the body comes from carbohydrates. This is because this is the only energy source that is stored as glycogen in your muscles. Without this energy source and its conversion in your muscles, athletes are unlikely to perform as well as they might otherwise be able to and they will also probably experience high levels of fatigue.

Given the amount of exercise that you do as an athlete, it is likely that the best diet for you is to observe the traditional balanced diet with plenty of fruits and vegetables. This should also include plenty of carbohydrates to sustain your volume of physical exertion. By incorporating some protein and whole foods and avoiding processed and junk foods you should still feel satisfied after meals and maintain a healthy weight and lifestyle.

If you are an athlete and you still wish to reduce your body fat percentage then it is recommended that you consult a nutritionist who specialises in sports nutrition. In this way they should be able to advise you so you can lose weight without compromising your performance.

HOW TO EAT LOW-CARB ON A BUDGET

If you're undertaking a new way of eating, such as a low-carb diet, you're probably wondering how your grocery bill will be affected. However, changing how you eat doesn't have to be a major monetary investment.

Buying more or less of specific foods, beverages, and other low-carb pantrystaples don't necessarily break the bank. Here are a few tips and tricks for eating low-carb on a budget.

Budget Basics

Even if you're not following a specific diet, being aware of the cost of groceries and trying to stick to a budget is a common experience for many shoppers. If you're on a low-carb diet, you'll also want to factor in the nutritional value of the foods you buy as well as eating a varied, balanced, diet.

Convenience, prep, and cooking requirements are also likely to influence your decisions when you're shopping and planning meals.

• The great news is that Atkins encourages the consumption of dietary fat and fattier cuts of meat are often the cheapest! So cuts like pork belly, 20% fat minced beef and chicken legs or thighs are much cheaper than pork chops, lean beef or skinless chicken breasts.

• Vegetables are great on Atkins and they are very often on sale in supermarkets. If so, buy in bulk and freeze the veg you don't use. I often buy a huge cauliflower when it's on offer and steam it all and then freeze the half I don't use. Then you can use the rest whether it's to make a cauli-pizza base, cauliflower cheese or adding to soups or stews.

• This is great for foods that are seasonal too, such as celeriac. This is a must in my house as I enjoy celeriac chips & mash; instead of starchier potato. So I buy it in season and freeze for when it's not available in my local supermarket.

• Local markets are also a great way to eat on a budget as they are often much cheaper than supermarkets, especially for meat, fish and fresh produce. So visit your local market, even if it's once a month, and stock up on essentials.

• Shop around! As well as your local market, try getting some of your shopping from stores like Aldi or Lidl. I've found their fruit & vegetable section to be excellent and much cheaper than the larger supermarkets. They also have great deals on low carb staples like flaxseeds and avocados.

• Buy frozen, if the vegetables you like are cheaper in their frozen form then go ahead. Just check the label as, unbelievably, some veg may have added sugar!

• Buy in bulk and portion your food into individual servings. This works well for great savings on protein like buying a whole side of salmon and then split into 8 or so servings and freeze. Much, much cheaper than buying individual portions.

• Eggs are a super food and so cheap! So stock up on free range eggs and you'll be getting a great source of protein and other nutrients for a fraction of the price of other protein rich foods.

• If you cook up double the portion size of your dinner-time meal then you'll have leftovers for lunch the next day which can save you ££s. It's much better to have a portion of low carb curry for your lunch, rather than a boring old sandwich!

• Don't feed the family any differently. Atkins friendly meals can be so tasty but just skip the starchy side from your plate. For instance, if you have pork belly with roasted veg, give yourself cheesy cauliflower instead of mashed potato that you may serve to the rest of the family.

LOW CARB DINING OUT STRATEGIES

Everybody likes going out to eat, and there are plenty of easy ways to enjoy a night out while staying true to your low carb goals. Regardless if you're on an Atkins plan or a similar keto diet, there are plenty of great options that are low in carbs and big in flavor. Both Atkins and keto activate your body's fat-burning metabolism by restricting carbs, so people following either diet will be looking for the same types of meal choices. If you're planning a night out, here are some keto friendly restaurants and menu picks:

Olive Garden

Topping off our list of keto restaurant options is the Italian staple, Olive Garden. If you are in the mood for seafood, we recommend the Herb-Grilled Salmon (460 calories, 28g total fat, 8g carbs, 4g fiber, and 43g protein). This fish filet is bursting with flavor as it is grilled to perfection and topped with garlic herb butter. It also comes with a side of delicious parmesan garlic broccoli. If fish isn't your thing, we recommend giving the tasty Parmesan-Crusted Zucchini (90 calories, 7g total fat, 5g carbs, 1g fiber, and 4g protein).

Chili's

Chili's, the home of flavorful Tex-Mex and American cuisine, is a great spot for something that isn't easily replicated at home. This bar and grill provides several options for those of us eating keto at restaurants. If you're in the mood for some Mexican flavors and spices, we recommend ordering the Chicken or Steak Fajitas (440/640 calories, 14/38g fat, 21/21g carbs, 3/3g fiber, and 59/55g protein) and enjoying without the tortillas or toppings. Instead of getting rice on the side, a double order of vegetables will be a great complement. We suggest boxing half of it to-go for lunch the next day to cut down on carbs. If you're not in the mood for Mexican on your night out, you're in luck! The House BBQ Ribs are another keto friendly option. A half rack of ribs without sauce will account for 720 calories, 53g total fat, 11g carbs, 1g fiber, and 49g protein.

Buffalo Wild Wings

Wings, beer, sports, and low carb choices. That's why Buffalo Wild Wings is one of our favorite keto restaurant options. Now, we can't recommend you grab a beer, but the snack size Traditional Wings with Medium Sauce (390 calories, 23g fat, 0g fiber, 1g carbs, and 44g protein) should do the trick! These wings will taste great while keeping you on pace to meet your keto goals. We also advise you to check out the BWW nutritional guides, as many other sauces and dry rubs are low in carbs!

Carrabba's

Get your Italian night on with another keto eating out option, Carrabba's. Our first choice would be the Tuscan Grilled Filet (590 calories, 44g total fat, less than 1g carbs, 0g fiber, and 47g protein). This juicy piece of meat is loaded with flavor while low in carbs. Another great option is the Pollo Rosa Maria (620 calories, 37g total fat, 4g carbs, 1g fiber, and 65g protein). Grilled chicken is stuffed with creamy fontina cheese and cured prosciutto, then topped with mushrooms and basil lemon butter. Make sure to get vegetables as a substitution to pasta on the side!

The Cheesecake Factory

A place filled with desserts can't possibly have low carb or keto restaurant options, can it? Of course, it can! The Cheesecake factory is a fantastic keto friendly restaurant. With several options to choose from, we recommend the Pan Seared Branzino with Lemon Butter (1130 calories, 93g fat, 22g carbs, 5g fiber, and 50g protein). This rich Mediterranean sea bass will hit the spot!

Red Robin

Red Robin is the home of fresh, fire-grilled burgers. Not only their food is packed and full of flavor, but it is also perfect for a keto or low carb lifestyle. The Wedgie™ Burger

(560 calories, 35g total fat, 22g carbs, 5g fiber, and 40g protein) is our go-to. This lettuce wrapped burger is topped with smoked bacon, house-made guacamole, tomatoes, and red onions. Who needs fries when your burger comes with a side salad? This meal is perfect for anyone trying to fulfill their Atkins or keto goals.

Red Lobster

If you're in the mood for some seafood on your night out, Red Lobster is a delicious keto restaurant option for you. The steamed Live Maine Lobster (440 calories, 34g fat, 0g carbs, 0g fiber, and 33g protein) has zero carbs (nice!) and is full of protein. If you're feeling surf & turf and are able to still meet your daily goals with some added carbs, you can't go wrong with The Rock Lobster & 12 of NY Strip Steak Combo (1,250 calories, 83g fat, 27g carbs, 4g fiber, and 97g protein).

A Few Tips For Going Keto At Restaurants:

Now that you know which keto friendly restaurants exist, it's time to get out and treat yourself. If you're going out for dinner at a restaurant that's not on this list, we have a few tips to keep in mind when eating out keto:

1. Plan ahead! If you're going out to eat, check the menu online ahead of time. You can also ask for nutrition information when you arrive. By law, restaurants must have that information available, making it easier than ever to make smart choices.

2. Meat and veggie options are your friends! These will typically be your best bet for lowcarb and protein-rich food.

3. Condiments like ketchup, BBQ sauce, and honey mustard tend to be high in sneaky carbs. If you need to add flavor, we recommend yellow mustard, ranch dressing, hot sauce, or butter.

4. Many entrées are served with a starch on the side, so opt for a side salad instead.

5. Don't be afraid to ask the waiter or waitress about keto friendly or low carb options!

ATKINS LOW CARB RECIPES

LOW CARB BREAKFAST RECIPES

Almond and Coconut Muffin in a Minute Recipe

Prep Time: 3 Minutes
Style:American
Cook Time: 1 Minutes
Phase: Phase 2

* Any adjustments made to the serving values will only update the ingredients of that recipe and not change the directions.
9.9g Protein, 19.2g Fat, 2.9g Fiber, 231.6kcalCalories, 3.7g Net Carbs.

INGREDIENTS
• 2 tablespoons Almond Meal Flour
• 1 teaspoon Coconut flour, high fiber
• 1 teaspoon Sucralose Based Sweetener (Sugar Substitute)

- 1/2 teaspoon Cinnamon
- 1/4 teaspoon Baking Powder (Straight Phosphate, Double Acting)
- 1/8 teaspoon Salt
- 1 large Egg
- 1 teaspoon Extra Virgin Olive Oil
- 1 tablespoon Sour Cream

DIRECTIONS

1. Place all dry ingredients in a coffee mug. Stir to combine.

2. Add the egg, oil, and sour cream. Stir until thoroughly combined.

3. Microwave for 1 minute. Use a knife if necessary to help remove the muffin from the cup, slice, butter, eat. For best results, eat immediately.

Note: Almond Meal from whole almonds is preferred for this recipe. Your MIM can be toasted once it's cooked and topped with cream cheese if you like. Replace the cinnamon with other spices, sugar-free syrup or 1/2 tsp unsweetened cocoa (net carb count will be .2g higher). Change the shape by making it in a bowl.

COOKING TIP: Try adding a small amount of almond or coconut extract to boost their flavors!

Almond Muffin in a Minute Recipe

Prep Time: 3 Minutes
Style:American
Cook Time: 1 Minutes
Phase: Phase 2

* Any adjustments made to the serving values will only update the ingredients of that recipe and not change the directions.
12.3g Protein, 23.5g Fat, 3.6g Fibre, 276.9kcalCalories, 4.5g Net Carbs.

INGREDIENTS
• 1/4 cup Bob's Red Mill Almond Meal/Flour (1/4 cup is 28g)
• 1 teaspoon No Calorie Sweetener
• 1/4 teaspoon Baking Powder (Straight Phosphate, Double Acting)
• 1 dash Salt
• 1/2 teaspoon Cinnamon
• 1 large Egg (Whole)
• 1 teaspoon Canola Vegetable Oil

DIRECTIONS

1. Place all dry ingredients in a coffee mug. Stir to combine.

2. Add the egg and oil. Stir until thoroughly combined.

3. Microwave for 1 minute. Use a knife if necessary to help remove the muffin from the cup, slice, butter, eat.

Note: Your MIM can be toasted once it's cooked and topped with cream cheese if you like. Replace the cinnamon with other spices, sugar-free syrup or 1/2 tsp unsweetened cocoa (net carb count will be .2g higher). Add a tablespoon of sour cream for a moister MIM. Change the shape by making it in a bowl.

COOKING TIP :Stirring the dry ingredients is a very important step to make sure your MIM bakes evenly.

Keto Almond Protein Pancakes

Prep Time: 5 Minutes
Style:American
Cook Time: 10 Minutes
Phase: Phase 2
Difficulty: Moderate

* Any adjustments made to the serving values will only update the ingredients of that recipe and not change the directions.
21.9g Protein, 9.1g Fat, 1.3g Fiber, 187.4kcalCalories, Net Carbs 3.2g.

INGREDIENTS
• 2 ounces Vanilla Whey Protein
• 1/4 cup Almond Meal Flour
• 3 tablespoons Whole Grain Soy Flour
• 1 teaspoon Baking Powder (Straight Phosphate, Double Acting)
• 3 large Eggs (Whole)
• 1/3 cup Large or Small Curd Creamed Cottage Cheese

DIRECTIONS
Top these naturally keto and low carb almond flour pancakes with almond butter, sugar-free syrup, or toasted almonds, if desired.

1. Mix the protein powder (1oz is about 4 Tbsp), almond meal, soy flour and baking powder together. Whisk the eggs, then blend together with the cottage cheese (substitute cream cheese if cottage cheese is not on your accepted foods list).

2. Heat a large nonstick skillet or griddle over medium heat. Lightly grease with butter or canola oil.

3. Using about 1/4 cup per pancake, drop batter onto the skillet. When bubbles begin to form in the middle of each pancake, turn over and cook another 2 minutes or until firm.

4. Repeat, keeping pancakes warm in the oven.

COOKING TIP: Add blueberries to the batter to add a fruit serving to this low carb breakfast or post workout meal (just pay attention to net carbs whenever you add ingredients).

Almond Protein Pancakes with Blueberries Recipe

Prep Time: 5 Minutes
Style:American
Cook Time: 10 Minutes
Phase: Phase 2
Difficulty: Moderate

* Any adjustments made to the serving values will only update the ingredients of that recipe and not change the directions.
24g Protein, 13.9g Fat, 4.1g Fiber, 256.5kcalCalories, Net Carbs 6.3g.

INGREDIENTS
• 2 tablespoons Blanched Almond Flour
• 3/4 large Egg (Whole)
• 1 1/2 tablespoons Whole Grain Soy Flour
• 1/4 teaspoon Baking Powder (Straight Phosphate, Double Acting)
• 1/2 ounce Large or Small Curd Creamed Cottage Cheese
• 2 tablespoons Vanilla Whey Protein
• 1/4 cup Fresh Blueberries

DIRECTIONS
1. Combine the almond flour, protein powder, soy flour and baking powder

together. Stir in the beaten egg and cottage cheese until blended.

2. Heat a large nonstick skillet or griddle over medium heat. Lightly grease with butter or canola oil.

3. Using about 1/4 cup per pancake, drop batter onto the skillet. When bubbles begin to form in the middle of each pancake, turn over and cook another 2 minutes or until firm.

4. Serve with blueberries Or add blueberries to the pancake batter before cooking.

COOKING TIP : Whether you're feeding a family or cooking for one, you can update the serving settings above to reveal the required amount of ingredients.

Almond Raspberry Smoothie Recipe

Prep Time: 5 Minutes
Style:American
Cook Time: Minutes
Phase: Phase 2
Difficulty: Easy

* Any adjustments made to the serving values will only update the ingredients of that recipe and not change the directions.
18.2g Protein, 13.7g Fat, 6.9g Fiber, 259.4kcalCalories, 10.3g Net Carbs.

INGREDIENTS
• 4 ounces Greek Yogurt - Plain (Container)
• 1/2 cup Red Raspberries
• 20 each wholes Blanched & Slivered almonds
• 1/2 cup Pure Almond Milk - Unsweetened Original

DIRECTIONS
Feel free to come up with your own combination of other berries and nuts for this protein-packed smoothie. If you use frozen raspberries, make sure they contain no added sugar.
Combine the yogurt, raspberries, almonds and almond milk in a blender and purée until smooth and creamy.

COOKING TIP: Whether you're feeding a family or cooking for one, you can update the serving settings above to reveal the required amount of ingredients.

Almond-Pineapple Smoothie Recipe

Prep Time: 5 Minutes
Style:American
Cook Time: Minutes
Phase: Phase 3
Difficulty: Easy

* Any adjustments made to the serving values will only update the ingredients of that recipe and not change the directions.
10.7g Protein, 17.3g Fat 3.9g Fiber 275.7kcalCalories, 16.1g Net Carbs.

INGREDIENTS
• 1/2 cup (8 fluid ounces) Plain Yogurt (Whole Milk)
• 2 1/2 ounces Pineapple

- 20 each wholes Blanched & Slivered almonds
- 1/2 cup pure almond milk - unsweetened original

DIRECTIONS

Feel free to substitute other fruits or nuts for the pineapple and/or almonds (about 20 whole almonds, 3 Tbsp slivered). Be sure to use fresh pineapple in this smoothie. Canned pineapple is swimming in sugar.

Combine the yogurt, pineapple, almonds and almond milk in a blender and purée until smooth and creamy.

COOKING TIP: Whether you're feeding a family or cooking for one, you can update the serving settings above to reveal the required amount of ingredients.

Belgian Waffles Recipe
Prep Time: 10 Minutes
Style:French
Cook Time: 10 Minutes
Phase: Phase 1
Difficulty: Moderate

* Any adjustments made to the serving values will only update the ingredients of that recipe and not change the directions.
7.5g Protein, 7.6g Fat 1.7g Fiber, 115.9kcalCalories, Net Carbs 3.7g.

INGREDIENTS
• 1 cup whole grain soy flour
• 2 tablespoons sucralose based sweetener (Sugar Substitute)
• 3 teaspoons baking powder (Sodium Aluminum Sulfate, Double Acting)
• 1/2 teaspoon salt
• 1/4 cup heavy cream
• 3 large eggs
• 1 tablespoon sugar free syrup
• 1/4 cup (8 fluid ounces) water

DIRECTIONS
1. Heat waffle iron. Whisk together soy flour, sugar substitute, baking powder and salt. Add cream, eggs and syrup and stir

until well blended (batter will be stiff). Add cold water 1 tablespoon at a time until batter is easily spoonable and spreadable, about the consistency of a thick pancake batter.

2. Spray waffle iron with oil spray. Place approximately 3 tablespoons of batter in center of a waffle iron. Cook according to manufacturer's instructions until crisp and dark golden brown. Repeat with remaining batter. Serve warm.

COOKING TIP: Whether you're feeding a family or cooking for one, you can update the serving settings above to reveal the required amount of ingredients.

Bell Pepper Rings Filled with Eggs and Mozzarella Recipe

Prep Time: 10 Minutes
Style:American
Cook Time: 10 Minutes
Phase: Phase 1
Difficulty: Easy

* Any adjustments made to the serving values will only update the ingredients of that recipe and not change the directions.
19.6g Protein, 20.9g Fat 1.6g Fiber 292.1kcalCalories, Net Carbs 4.7g .

INGREDIENTS
• 1/2 large (approx 3-3/4" long, 3" dia) Bell Peppers
• 2 large Eggs (Whole)
• 1 teaspoon Canola Vegetable Oil
• 1/4 cup shredded Mozzarella Cheese (Whole Milk)

DIRECTIONS
1. Cut bell pepper in half across the middle, then cut two 1-inch rings. Remove seeds and ribs. Note that any color bell pepper works well in this recipe.
2. Place rings in sauté pan with oil over medium-high heat. Place an egg in each ring and cook until desired doneness (do not flip).
3. Top eggs with cheese and, cover pan and cook 1 more minute until cheese has melted. Season to taste with salt and freshly ground black pepper.
4. Serve immediately

COOKING TIP: Whether you're feeding a family or cooking for one, you can update the serving settings above to reveal the required amount of ingredients.

Berry Delicious Protein Shake Smoothie

Prep Time: 10 Minutes
Style:American
Cook Time: 0 Minutes
Phase: Phase 2
Difficulty: Easy

* Any adjustments made to the serving values will only update the ingredients of that recipe and not change the directions.
18.2g Protein, 12.7g Fat 13.8g Fiber 255.7kcalCalories, 7.5g Net Carbs.

INGREDIENTS
• 1 each Atkins Strawberry Shake
• 1 tablespoon Chia Seeds
• 1/2 cup Raspberries, fresh
• 1/4 cup Cucumber, raw, sliced
• 1/4 cup Kroger Riced Cauliflower, frozen (85g per 3/4 cup)

DIRECTIONS

For best results use a chilled Atkins shake. Pour shake and chia seeds into a blender and let sit for 5 minutes. Add remaining ingredients and process until smooth.

Black Forest Protein Smoothie

Prep Time: 5 Minutes
Style:American
Cook Time: 0 Minutes
Phase: Phase 2
Difficulty: Easy

* Any adjustments made to the serving values will only update the ingredients of that recipe and not change the directions.
23.4g Protein, 5.7g Fat 2.6g Fiber 172.8kcalCalories, 6.7g Net Carbs.

INGREDIENTS
- 1/4 cup sweet cherries, frozen, unsweetened
- 1 cup coconut milk beverage, plain, unsweetened
- 1 scoop (1 scoop= 30 g) quest chocolate milkshake protein powder

DIRECTIONS

Blend all ingredients until very smooth. Pour over or blend with 1/2 cup of ice and enjoy.

Note that any sugar-free milk such as almond, soy or cashew may be substituted for the coconut.

COOKING TIP:Whether you're feeding a family or cooking for one, you can update the serving settings above to reveal the required amount of ingredients.

Blackberry Protein Smoothie Recipe

Prep Time: 5 Minutes
Style:American
Cook Time: 0 Minutes
Phase: Phase 2
Difficulty: Easy

* Any adjustments made to the serving values will only update the ingredients of that recipe and not change the directions.
16.5g Protein, 7.7g Fat, 8.1g Fiber 170.6kcalCalories, 7.2g Net Carbs.

INGREDIENTS
- 1/4 cup Blackberries, frozen, unsweetened
- 1 cup coconut milk beverage, plain, unsweetened
- 28 grams Atkins vanilla protein powder
- 1/8 teaspoon allspice, ground
- 1/8 teaspoon cinnamon, ground

DIRECTIONS
Blend all ingredients until very smooth. Pour over or blend with 1/2 cup of ice and enjoy.
Note that any sugar-free milk such as almond, soy or cashew may be sustituted for the coconut.

*28g = 1 scoop of Atkins Vanilla Protein Powder.

COOKING TIP: Whether you're feeding a family or cooking for one, you can update the serving settings above to reveal the required amount of ingredients.

Blackberry Smoothie Recipe

Prep Time: 5 Minutes
Style:American
Cook Time: 0 Minutes
Phase: Phase 2
Difficulty: Easy

* Any adjustments made to the serving values will only update the ingredients of that recipe and not change the directions.
25.3g Protein, 6.9g Fat, 5.2g Fiber, 209.7kcalCalories, 6.4g Net Carbs.

INGREDIENTS
• 1/4 cup frozen blackberries
• 1 cup coconut milk unsweetened
• 1 ounce vanilla whey protein
• 1 tablespoon organic 100% whole ground Golden flaxseed meal
• 1/4 teaspoon cinnamon
• 1/16 teaspoon allspice ground
• 1/2 teaspoon vanilla extract

DIRECTIONS
For this recipe unsweetened coconut, almond or soy milk may be used. Combine the frozen balckberries, milk of choice,

protein powder, flax meal, vanilla and spices in a blender. Blend until smooth.

COOKING TIP: To make a colder smoothie, try adding a couple ice cubes to the mix before blending!

Blueberry Scones Recipe

Prep Time: 15 Minutes
Style:French
Cook Time: 55 Minutes
Phase: Phase 2
Difficulty: Moderate

* Any adjustments made to the serving values will only update the ingredients of that recipe and not change the directions.
7.3g Protein, 18.2g Fat, 2.2g Fiber, 218.5kcalCalories, 6.3g Net Carbs.

INGREDIENTS
• 1 1/2 cups whole grain soy flour
• 3 tablespoons sucralose based sweetener (sugar substitute)
• 1 teaspoon salt
• 3 teaspoons baking powder (sodium aluminum sulfate, double acting)

- 6 tablespoons unsalted butter stick
- 2/3 cup heavy cream
- 1/4 cup sour cream
- 1 large egg
- 1 cup blueberries
- 2 teaspoons lemon zest

DIRECTIONS

1. In a food processor, pulse soy flour, sugar substitute, salt, and baking powder for 5 seconds, just to combine. Add butter and pulse until mixture resembles a coarse meal, about 30 seconds.

2. Pour into a large mixing bowl and toss with blueberries and lemon zest. In a large liquid measuring cup or small bowl, whisk heavy cream, sour cream and egg until well-mixed.

3. Chill the dough for 30 minutes. Preheat oven to 375°F. Separate dough into 10 equal-sized balls and pat each piece into a disk measuring 2 to 3 across. Space disks evenly on an ungreased baking sheet, leaving one inch between each scone.

4. Bake scones until bottoms are golden brown and tops are light golden. Cool on baking sheet set on a wire rack.

COOKING TIP: We love the idea of customizing this recipe to make it your own! If you add any ingredients, just be sure to keep an eye on net carbs.

Breakfast Mexi Peppers Recipe

Prep Time: 30 Minutes
Style:American
Cook Time: 30 Minutes
Phase: Phase 1
Difficulty: Moderate

* Any adjustments made to the serving values will only update the ingredients of that recipe and not change the directions.
18.9g Protein, 22.7g Fat, 1.5g Fiber
307.6kcalCalories, 5g Net Carbs.

INGREDIENTS
• 4 ounces pork and beef chorizo
• 4 ounces ground beef (80% Lean / 20% Fat)
• 1/2 cup chopped onions
• 1/4 cup shredded cheddar cheese
• 3 large eggs (Whole)
• 2 medium (approx 2-3/4" long, 2-1/2" diameter) sweet red peppers

DIRECTIONS

1. Preheat oven to 400°F. Line a baking sheet with foil.

2. Cook chorizo, stirring to break up lumps, until browned. Drain excess fat.

3. Place chorizo and ground beef in mixing bowl and combine with the onion, cheese and eggs.

4. Cut peppers in half lengthwise. Scoop out seeds and cut away ribs.

5. Fill each pepper with one-quarter of the meat mixture. Place on the prepared baking sheet. Bake for 25-30 minutes and serve hot.

COOKING TIP: Whether you're feeding a family or cooking for one, you can update the serving settings above to reveal the required amount of ingredients.

Breakfast Burrito recipe

Prep Time: 15 Minutes
Style:Mexican
Cook Time: 5 Minutes
Phase: Phase 2
Difficulty: Moderate

* Any adjustments made to the serving values will only update the ingredients of that recipe and not change the directions.
18.4g Protein, 20.1g Fat, 5.1g Fiber 287.5kcalCalories, 6.5g Net Carbs.

INGREDIENTS
• 4 large eggs (Whole)
• 1/2 teaspoon salt
• 1/4 teaspoon ror cayenne pepper
• 2 tortillas low carb tortillas
• 1 tablespoon canola vegetable oil
• 3 tablespoons sweet red peppers
• 2 tablespoons chopped ccallions or spring Onions
• 1 Jalapeno pepper
• 1/8 teaspoon tabasco sauce
• 2 ounces sauce

DIRECTIONS

1. Whisk eggs, salt and cayenne together in a bowl.

2. In a medium skillet over medium heat, toast tortillas 1 minute per side until brown in spots; set aside and cover with foil to keep warm. Dice the red pepper, scallions (separate the white from the green parts) and finely dice the jalapeno.

3. In the same skillet add oil, red pepper, scallion whites and jalapeno. Cook until vegetables are softened, about 3 minutes.

4. Add eggs and continue to cook, stirring, until eggs are set, about 2 minutes.

5. Place tortillas on plates. Divide eggs between tortillas, season with hot sauce and gently roll up.

6. Serve with salsa and scallion greens.

Note: This can be made with a whole wheat or low-carb tortilla if you are in an acceptable phase. The whole wheat tortillas used here have 20g NC each so be sure to adjust the NC to the tortilla you are using. Low-carb tortillas typically have less NC than the whole wheat.

COOKING TIP: Whether you're feeding a family or cooking for one, you can update the serving settings above to reveal the required amount of ingredients.

Breakfast Berry Parfait Recipe

Prep Time: 15 Minutes
Style:American
Cook Time: 0 Minutes
Phase: Phase 2
Difficulty: Moderate

* Any adjustments made to the serving values will only update the ingredients of that recipe and not change the directions.
10.3g Protein, 25.3g Fat, 7.6g Fiber, 339.6kcalCalories, 11g Net Carbs.

INGREDIENTS
• 1 1/2 cup, wholes strawberries
• 2 cups raspberries
• 2 1/2 tablespoons sucralose based sweetener (sugar substitute)
• 1 cup heavy cream
• 1 tablespoon vanilla extract
• 6 ounces greek yogurt - plain (container)

• 1 each Atkins almond coconut bar

DIRECTIONS
1. In a blender, purée 1 1/2 cups of the strawberries and 1 1/2 cups of the raspberries with 1 1/2 tablespoons sugar substitute. Chop the remaining 1/2 cup raspberries and fold into the puree.
2. In a large mixing bowl, with an electric mixer on medium speed, combine heavy cream, the remaining 1 tablespoon sugar substitute and the vanilla, beating to soft peaks. Add yogurt (1 1/2 single-serving containers) and beat to stiff peaks.
3. In four parfait glasses, alternate layers of the berry mixture, cream filling and crumbled Atkins bar, making at least two layers of each.
4. Top each with some of the remaining 1/2 cup strawberries and serve.

COOKING TIP: Whether you're feeding a family or cooking for one, you can update the serving settings above to reveal the required amount of ingredients.

Blueberry, Maple and Pecan Smoothie Recipe
Prep Time: 5 Minutes
Style:American
Cook Time: 0 Minutes
Phase: Phase 2
Difficulty: Easy

* Any adjustments made to the serving values will only update the ingredients of that recipe and not change the directions.
26.6g Protein, 15.3g Fat, 3.3g Fiber, 281.8kcalCalories, 9.6g Net Carbs.

INGREDIENTS
• 1/4 cup blueberries, fresh
• 10 each pecan Halves, raw
• 1 cup coconut milk beverage, plain, unsweetened
• 1 scoop (1 scoop= 31 g) quest vanilla milkshake protein powder
• 1 tablespoon maple syrup (sugar-free)
• 1 tablespoon lemon juice

DIRECTIONS

Blend all ingredients except ice until very smooth. Pour over or blend with 1/2 cup of ice and enjoy.

Note that any sugar-free milk such as almond, soy or cashew may be sustituted for the coconut.

COOKING TIP: Why not have friends over to enjoy this drink! Update the serving settings above to reveal the required amount of ingredients you'll need.

Breakfast Sausage Sautéed with Red and Green Bell Peppers Recipe

Prep Time: 5 Minutes
Style:Other
Cook Time: 10 Minutes
Phase: Phase 1
Difficulty: Easy

* Any adjustments made to the serving values will only update the ingredients of that recipe and not change the directions.
29.8g Protein, 20.9g Fat, 1.5g Fiber, 328.4kcalCalories, 3.1g Net Carbs.
INGREDIENTS

- 1 teaspoon canola vegetable oil
- 4 link, cookeds turkey breakfast sausage
- 1/4 large (2.25 per pound, approx 3-3/4" long, 3" diameter) red sweet pepper
- 1/4 large (2.25 per pound, approx 3-3/4" long, 3" diameter) green sweet pepper
- 1 slice (1 ounce) monterey jack cheese

DIRECTIONS

1. Heat a skillet with 1 teaspoon oil over medium-high heat.

2. Crumble the sausage link or leave whole and slice after cooking. Sauté until just beginning to brown. About 3 minutes. Dice the peppers and add them to the sausage. Cook until sausage is browned and peppers are softened, about 5 minutes.

3. Sprinkle cheese on top and allow to melt 1-2 minutes. Serve immediately.

COOKING TIP: Whether you're feeding a family or cooking for one, you can update the serving settings above to reveal the required amount of ingredients.

Broccolini and Bacon Egg Bites Recipe

Prep Time: 5 Minutes
Style:American
Cook Time: 40 Minutes
Phase: Phase 1
Difficulty: Moderate

* Any adjustments made to the serving values will only update the ingredients of that recipe and not change the directions.
14.8g Protein, 23.1g Fat, 0.3g Fiber, 282.6kcalCalories, 3.4g Net Carbs.

 INGREDIENTS
• 8 servings olive oil palm (0.5g = 0.6sec spray)
• 5 slices bacon
• 6 stalks broccolini, fresh, steamed
• 5 each egg
• 6 tablespoons cream cheese, original
• 1 ounce feta cheese
• 3 teaspoons hot sauce - cholula hot sauce
• 1/2 teaspoon(s) kosher salt (1/4 tsp= 1.5 g)
• 1 1/2 cups arugula, raw
• 1 tablespoon lemon juice
• 1 tablespoon olive oil
• 1/8 teaspoon black pepper, ground

DIRECTIONS

Preheat the oven to 350°F. Lightly coat eight silicone egg-bite mold cups or eight cups of a standard nonstick muffin tin with cooking spray, or line a regular (not nonstick) muffin tin with nonstick muffin liners and set into a large baking pan.

In a large nonstick skillet, cook the bacon over medium heat until golden, about 5 minutes per side. Transfer to a paper towel-lined plate to drain. Chop the bacon into small pieces.

Meanwhile, in a blender, puree the eggs, cream cheese, feta cheese, hot sauce, and 1/4 teaspoon salt until smooth.

Pour off all but 1 tablespoon of fat from the skillet. Add the broccolini, 1 tablespoon water, and 1/4 teaspoon salt. Cook over medium-high heat, stirring frequently, until the broccolini is tender, 3 to 5 minutes. Remove from the heat.

Fill each of the egg cups with 1 heaping teaspoon of bacon and one heaping tablespoon of broccolini. Top with the egg mixture, filling the cups to about 1 inch from the top (you may have a bit left over; discard or saute in a skillet for a mini snack). Add just enough boiled water to the baking pan to come halfway up the sides of the molds.

Bake the egg bites until set, 20 to 25 minutes. Take the pan from the oven, then take the molds from the water bath. Let the egg bites cool for a few minutes, then take them from the molds.

In a medium bowl, toss together the arugula, lemon juice, oil, and a pinch each of salt and pepper. Place 3/4 cup of salad and 2 egg bites on each of four plates and serve.

Adapt this recipe for Atkins 40 by adding 1/4 cup fresh blueberries per serving
Adapt this recipe for Atkins 100 by adding 1 slice toasted Ezekiel sprouted grain bread per serving

COOKING TIP: This and 50 other delicious and adaptable recipes can be found in The Atkins 100 Eating Solution, Easy Low-Carb Living for Everyday Wellness

LOW CARB DINNER & ENTRÉE RECIPES

Nachos Stuffed Chicken Breast Recipe

Prep Time: 25 Minutes
Style:Mexican
Cook Time: 25 Minutes
Phase: Phase 1
Difficulty: Moderate

* Any adjustments made to the serving values will only update the ingredients of that recipe and not change the directions.
79.5g Protein, 31.6g Fat, 1.8g Fiber, 650.1kcalCalories, 6.8g Net Carbs.

INGREDIENTS
• 4 ounces cabot pepper jack cheese
• 1/3 cup sour cream
• 1 medium (4-1/8" long) scallions, raw
• 2 tablespoons cilantro, fresh, chopped
• 1 3/4 teaspoon(s) Kosher salt (1/4 tsp= 1.5 g)
• 32 ounces chicken breast filet, skinless
• 2 teaspoons chili powder

- 2 servings olive oil pam (0.5g = 0.6sec spray)
- 1 each tomato, medium 4.6 oz
- 4 tablespoons lime juice
- 3 tablespoons olive oil
- 1/2 teaspoon erythritol
- 1/8 teaspoon black pepper, ground
- 5 cup (47.3g) mixed baby greens

DIRECTIONS

Preheat the oven to 400°F.

In a small bowl, combine the cheese, sour cream, scallion, cilantro, and 1/2 teaspoon salt.

Insert a small sharp knife into the thickest part of each chicken breast and push it three-quarters of the way down to the thin end, being careful not to pierce the outside of the breast. Move the knife from side to side to form a wide pocket with a opening.

Stuff each breast with a quarter of the cheese mixture (about 1/4 cup). Secure with toothpicks. Season the chicken with the chili powder and 1 teaspoon salt.

Lightly coat a large ovenproof skillet with cooking spray and heat over medium-high heat until hot but not smoking. Place the chicken breasts into the skillet and cook until golden, about 2 minutes per side.

Transfer the skillet to the oven and roast until an instant-read thermometer inserted into the thickest part of the breast reads 165°F, 18 to 20 minutes.

Meanwhile, prepare the dressing: in a small bowl, whisk the lime juice, oil, erythritol, and a generous pinch each of salt and pepper together until combined.

Remove the chicken from the oven. Remove and discard the toothpicks, then arrange the chicken on four serving plates. Mound 1 1/4 cups greens alongside each chicken breast, then drizzle the greens with about 1 1/2 tablespoons of dressing per serving. Top each portion with 2 heaping tablespoons of chopped tomato and cilantro to taste and serve.

Adapt for Atkins 40 by serving with 2 tablespoons canned refried black beans per serving

Adapt for Atkins 100 by serving with ½ cup canned refried black beans per serving

COOKING TIP: This and 50 other delicious and adaptable recipes can be found in The Atkins 100 Eating Solution, Easy Low-Carb Living for Everyday Wellness.

Acorn Squash with Spiced Applesauce and Maple Drizzle Recipe

Prep Time: 8 Minutes
Style:American
Cook Time: 20 Minutes
Phase: Phase 3
Difficulty: Moderate

* Any adjustments made to the serving values will only update the ingredients of that recipe and not change the directions.
0.7g Protein, 3.3g Fat, 2.2g Fiber, 72.8kcalCalories, 9.7g Net Carbs.

INGREDIENTS
• 1 squash (4 inch diameter) acorn winter squash
• 5 teaspoons unsalted butter stick
• 1/2 teaspoon salt
• 1/2 teaspoon black pepper
• 3/4 cup applesauce (without added ascorbic acid, unsweetened, canned)
• 1/8 teaspoon cinnamon
• 1 tablespoon sugar free maple flavored syrup

DIRECTIONS

1. Preheat oven to 350°F. Cut squash in half, remove seeds and then cut into 6 wedges.

2. Line a sheet pan with aluminum foil. Melt 1 tablespoon (3 teaspoons) butter and brush on squash; sprinkle with salt and pepper. Place on pan and bake until squash is fork tender, about 20 minutes.

3. In a small pot heat the applesauce, about 3 minutes. Stir in 2 teaspoons butter and cinnamon and cook 30 seconds more.

4. Serve squash with a dollop of applesauce mixture and a drizzle of syrup (about 1/2 teaspoon each).

COOKING TIP: Having a party? When planning your low carb spread, think about which dishes you can make in advance and which need fresh ingredients that day.

Air-Fryer One Pot Chicken and Vegetables

Prep Time: 10 Minutes
Style:American
Cook Time: 25 Minutes
Phase: Phase 4
Difficulty: Easy

* Any adjustments made to the serving values will only update the ingredients of that recipe and not change the directions.
46.1g Protein, 45.5g Fat, 6.2g Fiber, 709.6kcalCalories, Net Carbs 20.8g.

INGREDIENTS
• 6 ounces chicken thigh, boneless, with skin
• 1/2 sweetpotato, 5" long sweet potato
• 4 teaspoons ghee
• 1/4 teaspoon Salt
• 1/4 teaspoon Black Pepper, ground
• 1 cup Red Cabbage, steamed, shredded
• 1/8 tablespoon apple cider vinegar
• 1/8 teaspoon cayenne pepper
• 1/16 teaspoon (3.5g) truvia
• 1/16 teaspoon Chili powder
• 1/16 teaspoon garlic powder
• 1/16 teaspoon paprika

DIRECTIONS

1. Preheat air fryer to 375°F for at least 3 minutes. Season both sides of the chicken thigh with salt and pepper, and cook skin side down in the air fryer alone for 12 minutes.

2. While the chicken begins to cook, cut the sweet potato into ½-inch julienne, or French fry shape. Toss with 1 tablespoon melted ghee, 1/8 teaspoon salt and 1/8 teaspoon pepper.

3. When the chicken has reached the 12 minute mark, turn it over and add the sweet potato fries to the air fryer in a single layer. Continue to cook for 5 minutes.

4. While the sweet potatoes and chicken cook, slice two 1-inch thick "steaks" from the cabbage. Spread each side of each cabbage slice with ½ teaspoon ghee and season with a pinch of salt and pepper. After 5 minutes of cooking the sweet potatoes and chicken, shake the fryer basket to toss the sweet potatoes, and add the cabbage on top of the chicken and sweet potatoes. Cook all the components for another 8 minutes.

5. While the cooking completes, combine the vinegar with 1 teaspoon ghee, cayenne, stevia and erythritol sweetener, chili

powder, garlic, and paprika in a small bowl. This recipe gives a medium level of spice. If you prefer your chicken more spicy, you can double the amount of cayenne.

6. Remove the cabbage and sweet potatoes from the air fryer to a plate. Check the chicken for doneness using an instant read thermometer to ensure an internal temperature of 165°. Remove the fully cooked chicken from the air fryer and spread each side of the chicken with half of the spicy oil.

Keto Alfredo Sauce Recipe

Prep Time: 20 Minutes
Style:Italian
Cook Time: 0 Minutes
Phase: Phase 1
Difficulty: Easy

* Any adjustments made to the serving values will only update the ingredients of that recipe and not change the directions.
10.5g Protein, 33.3g Fat, 0g Fiber, 348.6kcalCalories, 2.7g Net Carbs.

INGREDIENTS
- 2 tablespoons unsalted butter stick
- 1 1/2 cups heavy cream
- 1/2 cup parmesan cheese (trated)
- 4 ounces romano cheese
- 1/8 teaspoon black pepper
- 1/8 teaspoon nutmeg (Ground)

DIRECTIONS
One of the simplest and best of all pasta sauces, Alfredo sauce is versatile enough to dress up steamed vegetables as well. For the best flavor, buy blocks of Parmesan and Pecorino Romano and grate them yourself. See a variation below. Each serving is 1/4 cup.

1. Melt butter in a medium saucepan over medium heat. Add cream and simmer until reduced to 1 cup, about 10 minutes. Grate Parmesan and Romano cheeses.
2. Remove from heat; stir in Parmesan, Romano, pepper and nutmeg until the cheeses have melted and sauce is smooth.
3. Serve immediately.
Vodka Sauce: Prepare Alfredo Sauce according   to   directions,   adding   3

tablespoons tomato paste and 2 tablespoons vodka to the heavy cream before reducing.
COOKING TIP: Alfredo sauce on zoodles are delish! Try our Zucchini Chicken Alfredo recipe.

Nachos Stuffed Chicken Breast Recipe

Prep Time: 25 Minutes
Style:Mexican
Cook Time: 25 Minutes
Phase: Phase 1
Difficulty: Moderate

* Any adjustments made to the serving values will only update the ingredients of that recipe and not change the directions.
79.5g Protein, 31.6g Fat, 1.8g Fiber, 650.1kcalCalories, 6.8g Net Carbs.

INGREDIENTS
- 4 ounces cabot pepper jack cheese
- 1/3 cup sour cream
- 1 medium (4-1/8" long) scallions, raw
- 2 tablespoons Cilantro, fresh, chopped
- 1 3/4 teaspoon(s) Kosher salt (1/4 tsp= 1.5 g)

- 32 ounces chicken breast filet, skinless
- 2 teaspoons chili powder
- 2 servings olive oil Pam (0.5g = 0.6sec spray)
- 1 each Tomato, medium 4.6 oz
- 4 tablespoons lime juice
- 3 tablespoons olive oil
- 1/2 teaspoon erythritol
- 1/8 teaspoon black pepper, ground
- 5 cup (47.3g) mixed baby greens

DIRECTIONS

Preheat the oven to 400°F.

In a small bowl, combine the cheese, sour cream, scallion, cilantro, and 1/2 teaspoon salt.

Insert a small sharp knife into the thickest part of each chicken breast and push it three-quarters of the way down to the thin end, being careful not to pierce the outside of the breast. Move the knife from side to side to form a wide pocket with a opening. Stuff each breast with a quarter of the cheese mixture (about 1/4 cup). Secure with toothpicks. Season the chicken with the chili powder and 1 teaspoon salt.

Lightly coat a large ovenproof skillet with cooking spray and heat over medium-high heat until hot but not smoking. Place the chicken breasts into the skillet and cook until golden, about 2 minutes per side. Transfer the skillet to the oven and roast until an instant-read thermometer inserted into the thickest part of the breast reads 165°F, 18 to 20 minutes.

Meanwhile, prepare the dressing: in a small bowl, whisk the lime juice, oil, erythritol, and a generous pinch each of salt and pepper together until combined.

Remove the chicken from the oven. Remove and discard the toothpicks, then arrange the chicken on four serving plates. Mound 1 1/4 cups greens alongside each chicken breast, then drizzle the greens with about 1 1/2 tablespoons of dressing per serving. Top each portion with 2 heaping tablespoons of chopped tomato and cilantro to taste and serve.

Adapt for Atkins 40 by serving with 2 tablespoons canned refried black beans per serving

Adapt for Atkins 100 by serving with ½ cup canned refried black beans per serving

COOKING TIP: This and 50 other delicious and adaptable recipes can be found in The

Atkins 100 Eating Solution, Easy Low-Carb
Living for Everyday Wellness.

LOW CARB SNACK RECIPES

Keto Air Fryer Jalapeno Poppers

Prep Time: 20 Minutes
Style:American
Cook Time: 15 Minutes
Phase: Phase 1
Difficulty: Easy

* Any adjustments made to the serving values will only update the ingredients of that recipe and not change the directions.
3.3g Protein, 5.9g Fat, 0.6g Fiber, 71.7kcalCalories, 1.1g Net Carbs-

INGREDIENTS
• 7 tablespoons cream cheese, original
• 1/4 cup shredded cheddar cheese
• 1/4 cup shredded monterey cheese
• 1/2 teaspoon chili powder
• 240 Jalapeno peppers
• 6 slices bacon

Ingredient note: 240 grams of jalapenos is equivalent to 6 (3-4-inch) jalapenos.

DIRECTIONS

1. Heat air fryer to 390°F.

2. In a small bowl, combine the cream cheese, cheddar, Monterey jack, and chili powder until well combined and evenly distributed.

3. Slice each jalapeno in half lengthwise. Use a spoon to scoop out the seeds and discard, then fill with cream cheese mix (do not overfill). Slice the bacon in half, and loosely drape a slice of bacon over each filled jalapeno, securing the bacon on the top and bottom with a toothpick or skewer.

4. Cook, in batches if needed, for 6 minutes, or until the bacon is crispy and the cheese has melted. Remove from air fryer and serve.

COOKING TIP: This naturally keto and low carb recipe is a great for sharing!

Asian Chicken Handrolls with Peanut Sauce Recipe

Prep Time: 0 Minutes
Style:Asian
Cook Time: 0 Minutes
Phase: Phase 2
Difficulty: Difficult

* Any adjustments made to the serving values will only update the ingredients of that recipe and not change the directions.
33.9g Protein, 23.9g Fat, 7.3g Fiber, 414kcalCalories, 8.3g Net Carbs.

INGREDIENTS
• 8 ounces chicken yenderloins
• 1 1/2 tablespoons organic tamari
• 1 tablespoon rice vinegar
• 1 teaspoon ginger
• 1 serving liquid Stevia
• 1/2 avocado, florida or californium Avocados
• 1/4 cucumber (8-1/4") Cucumber (with Peel)
• 2 1/2 ounces yambean (Jicama)
• 8 sprigs cilantro
• 2 sheets sushi nori roasted seaweed
• 1/2 tablespoon vegetable oil

- 1 1/2 servings 100% natural creamy Peanut Butter
- 4 tablespoons tap water
- 3/4 teaspoon sriracha chili sauce

DIRECTIONS

1. Marinate the chicken tenderloins by placing them in a plastic bag with 1 tbsp tamari, 1 tbsp rice vinegar, 1/2 tsp minced ginger and 3-4 drops stevia. Set aside.

2. While the chicken marinates prepare the vegetables. Slice the avocado into 8 long pieces. Cut the cucumber and jicama into sticks measuring about 3 x 1/8 inches. Divide ingredients into 4 equal sets. Set all aside on a cutting board along with the sprigs of cilantro. Gently fold the nori sheets in half and then rip them in two, set all 4 sheets aside.

3. Place the vegetable oil in a nonstick skillet over medium-high heat. Add the chicken, discarding the remaining marinade and plastic bag. Cook until no longer pink in the center; about 3 minutes per side. Place on the cutting board with the other ingredients and slice each tenderloin into 3 pieces (if you only had 3 tenderloins, cut into an amount that is easily divided by 4).

Place a small dish of water next to the assembly line. Set aside.

4. In a small bowl combine the peanut butter, water, 1 1/2 tsp tamari, 1/2 tsp minced ginger, 3-4 drops stevia and 3/4 tsp sriracha. Blend until all ingredients are incorporated, adjust seasonings to your taste by adding more tamari, ginger, stevia or sriracha.

5. Assembly: Place the 1/2 sheet of nori on a flat surface. Place the sliced avocado, cucumber, jicama, and cilantro at a slight angle so they align with the corner of one end of the nori sheet with about 1/2-inch of the corner of the nori sheet sticking out. Dredge the chicken in the peanut sauce and place it on top of the vegetables. Roll, starting at the side where you placed the ingredients, then change direction slightly so that it creates a cone shape with one end rolling tightly and the other end open. With your finger tips, dip them in the water bowl, and add water to the nori sheet on the end corner of the wrap, hold it down a few seconds to seal the wrap in place. Repeat for remaining wraps.

6. Serve wraps with any remaining sauce for dipping.

COOKING TIP: Whether you're feeding a family or cooking for one, you can update the serving settings above to reveal the required amount of ingredients.

Air Fryer Korean Chicken Wings

Prep Time: 250 Minutes
Style:Asian
Cook Time: 30 Minutes
Phase: Phase 1
Difficulty: Easy

* Any adjustments made to the serving values will only update the ingredients of that recipe and not change the directions.
17.7g Protein, 21.5g Fat, 1.4g Fiber, 291.5kcalCalories, 1.7g Net Carbs.

INGREDIENTS
• 1/2 cup kimchi kraut juice
• 1 cup buttermilk, whole milk
• 4 tablespoons sambal oelek ground fresh Chili Paste
• 1 each egg
• 2 each garlic, clove
• 1 teaspoon salt
• 1 teaspoon black pepper, ground

- 2 pounds chicken wing, meat and skin, raw
- 1/2 cup kimchi, cabbage
- 8 tablespoons mayonnaise (Hellman's Real)
- 6 teaspoons sriracha hot sauce (Rooster sauce)

DIRECTIONS

1. Using a fine mesh strainer collect ½ cup juice from the kimchi. Use a clean kitchen towel and squeeze the kimchi to release more juice if needed. Mince or press the garlic. In a small bowl, use a fork to whisk together the kimchi juice, buttermilk, red chili paste, egg, garlic, salt, and pepper.

2. Place the chicken wings in a zipper-lock freezer bag, pour in the buttermilk mixture, and toss to coat. Place in the refrigerator to marinate for at least 4 hours or overnight, turning at least a few times to ensure even coating with the marinade.

3. Preheat your air fryer to 390°F for about 10 minutes.

4. Place the chicken in a single layer in the warm Air Fryer and cook for 9-10 minutes for drumettes, 7-8 minutes for wings, or until chicken reaches an internal temperature of 165°F, turning once in the middle of the

cooking time. Complete this step in batches if needed.

5. In a food processor, chop the strained and squeezed out kimchi until it is fine pieces. Add the mayonnaise and Sriracha and process until it is the consistency of tartar sauce. Serve alongside the chicken wings as a dipping sauce. One serving is about 2 wings and 1 ½ tablespoons dipping sauce.

NOTE: Because only about about 30% of the marinade is likely to be consumed, corrected nutritionals per serving for this recipe are as follows: Total carbs- 2.15; Net carbs- 1.67; Protein- 16.44; Fiber- 0.48; Fat- 20.18; Calories- 260.9

Air Fryer Pepperoni Chips Recip

Prep Time: 0 Minutes
Style:Italian
Cook Time: 4 Minutes
Phase: Phase 1
Difficulty: Easy

* Any adjustments made to the serving values will only update the ingredients of that recipe and not change the directions. 5.7g Protein, 11.3g Fat, 0.4g Fiber, 130.5kcalCalories, 0.7g Net Carbs.

INGREDIENTS
• 56 grams Pepperoni
Ingredient Notes: We used 3-inch diameter pepperoni slices that are ¼-ounce each. Changing the size and thickness of the pepperoni will change the optimal cooking time.

DIRECTIONS
1. Preheat your air fryer to 390°F for at least 3 minutes.
2. Create a single layer with only minimal overlap of pepperoni on the fryer plate. Cover with the dehydrator rack to help keep

the pepperoni in place. Fry for 3 minutes 30 seconds.

3. Remove pepperoni slices from the air fryer and allow to cool on a paper towel lined plate for at least 1 minute. Repeat steps 2 and 3 if needed to fry all the pepperoni slices.

4. These chips can be eaten as is, or dipped in guacamole for a delicious snack!

Apple Muffins with Cinnamon-Pecan Streusel Recipe

Prep Time: 15 Minutes
Style:American
Cook Time: 25 Minutes
Phase: Phase 3
Difficulty: Moderate

* Any adjustments made to the serving values will only update the ingredients of that recipe and not change the directions.
7.6g Protein, 21.1g Fat, 5.1g Fiber, 246.6kcalCalories, 5.2g Net Carbs.

INGREDIENTS
- 1 2/3 cups almond meal flour
- 1/2 cup, half pecans
- 6 1/2 teaspoons cinnamon
- 1/3 teaspoon salt
- 6 tablespoons erythritol
- 1/16 pinch stevia
- 2 tablespoons unsalted butter stick
- 2 large eggs (Whole)
- 1/4 cup coconut milk unsweetened
- 2 teaspoons vanilla extract
- 2 tablespoons organic high fiber coconut Flour
- 1 teaspoon baking powder (Straight Phosphate, Double Acting)
- 2/3 cup, quartered or chopped apple

DIRECTIONS
1. Preheat oven to 350 F. Prepare a muffin tin with 8 cupcake papers.
2. Combine 2/3 cup almond flour, chopped pecans, 2 tablespoons cinnamon, 1/8 teaspoon salt, 2 tablespoons granular sugar substitute (eryhtritol), a pinch of stevia and 2 tablespoons melted butter in a small bowl. Mix with a fork until it begins to crumble. Set aside while making the muffin batter.
3. For the muffins: whisk together the eggs, 1/4 cup coconut milk, 2 teaspoons vanilla, 6

tablespoons granular sugar substitute (erythritol), a pinch of stevia, and 1/2 teaspoon ground cinnamon. Add 1 cup almond flour, 2 tablespoons coconut flour, 1/4 teaspoon salt and 1 teaspoon baking powder; mix to combine then fold in 2/3 cup finely chopped apples.

4. Divide into muffin 8 wells topping each with about 2 tablespoons of the struesal. Bake for 25 minutes, remove from oven and allow to sit for 10-20 minutes to cool before removing. These may be eaten immediately or stored in an airtight container in the refrigerator for up to 1 week.

COOKING TIP: We love the idea of customizing this recipe to make it your own! If you add any ingredients, just be sure to keep an eye on net carbs.

Atkins Mini Muffins Recipe

Prep Time: 10 Minutes
Style:American
Cook Time: 25 Minutes
Phase: Phase 3
Difficulty: Moderate

* Any adjustments made to the serving values will only update the ingredients of that recipe and not change the directions.
5.6g Protein, 4.4g Fat, 0.8g Fiber, 71.5kcalCalories, 2.1g Net Carbs.

INGREDIENTS
• 3 teaspoons baking powder (Straight Phosphate, Double Acting)
• 1/3 cup sucralose based sweetener (Sugar Substitute)
• 2 tablespoons unsalted butter stick
• 1 cup sour cream (Cultured)
• 2 large eggs (Whole)
• 6 servings Atkins flour mix

DIRECTIONS

Use the Atkins recipe to make Atkins Flour Mix for this recipe, you will need 2 cups.

1. Preheat oven to 350°F.

2. Blend all dry ingredients together in a large mixing bowl. Then add wet ingredients with a spoon or spatula and mix thoroughly.

3. Lightly coat mini muffin tins with non-stick vegetable oil spray (or use paper mini muffin cups).

4. Spoon dough mixture into mini muffin tins and bake for 18-22 minutes or until done. Recipe makes 24 mini muffins. *Add berries if desired but remember to account for additional Net Carbs.

COOKING TIP: Whether you're feeding a family or cooking for one, you can update the serving settings above to reveal the required amount of ingredients.

Baked Goat Cheese and Ricotta Custards Recipe
Prep Time: 0 Minutes
Style:Italian
Cook Time: 50 Minutes
Phase: Phase 2
Difficulty: Moderate

* Any adjustments made to the serving values will only update the ingredients of that recipe and not change the directions.
22.4g Protein, 27.8g Fat, 1.1g Fiber, 356.6kcalCalories, 4.1g Net Carbs

INGREDIENTS
- 1 cup ricotta cheese (Whole Milk)
- 6 ounces goats cheese (Semisoft)
- 3 tablespoons parmesan cheese (Grated)
- 1/4 cup chopped english walnuts
- 2 tablespoons basil
- 2 large eggs (Whole)
- 1/8 teaspoon Salt
- 1/8 teaspoon black pepper
- 12 leaves spinach

DIRECTIONS

This recipe is suitable for all phases except the first two weeks of Induction due ot the nuts.

1. Heat oven to 350°F. Spray cooking spray onto four 5-ounce ramekins or custard cups.

2. Combine ricotta, goat cheese, Parmesan, walnuts, basil, egg, salt, and pepper in a bowl and mix well.

3. Line each ramekin with 3 spinach leaves. Divide cheese mixture; fill full. Bake 30 minutes. Cool 5 minutes.

4. To serve, run a knife around the rim of each custard. Invert onto small plates. Season with salt and pepper to taste.

Note: Photo shown includes Atkins Pie Crust which contains gluten and is not suitable until Phase 3. Follow link to recipe, make full recipe, rolling out just enough to fill mini muffin tins with the custard recipe above. Prebake the crusts for 8 min then fill and bake another 30 minutes. You will have some leftover crust - simply form into a disk and freeze for another use.

COOKING TIP: Having a party? When planning your low carb spread, think about which dishes you can make in advance and which need fresh ingredients that day.

LOW CARB APPETIZERS & SIDE DISH RECIPES

Artichokes with Lemon-Butter Recipe

Prep Time: 10 Minutes
Style:Other
Cook Time: 15 Minutes
Phase: Phase 1
Difficulty: Easy

* Any adjustments made to the serving values will only update the ingredients of that recipe and not change the directions.
5.4g Protein, 23.8g Fat 9.6g Fiber, 287.9kcalCalories, 10.7g Net Carbs.

INGREDIENTS
• 4 artichoke, media Artichokes (Globe or French)
• 4 fruit (2-1/8" diameter) Lemon
• 2 tablespoons coriander seed
• 2 tablespoons salt
• 1/2 cup unsalted butter stick

DIRECTIONS

1. Bring 4 quarts of water to a boil in a large pot. Trim the stems of the artichokes to about 2 inches.

2. Halve 3 lemons and squeeze juice into water. Add lemon halves, coriander seeds and salt. Place artichokes in the cooking liquid, and cover with a heavy plate to keep them from floating. Boil 15 minutes, until a paring knife, inserted where the stem meets the bottom, comes out easily. Remove and drain excess water.

3. In a small bowl, melt butter in a microwave or saucepan. Mix in juice of remaining lemon, salt and pepper.

4. Serve each person one whole artichoke, accompanied by a ramekin of butter sauce and a large bowl for discarded leaves. Season with freshly ground salt and pepper to taste.

COOKING TIP: Having a party? When planning your low carb spread, think about which dishes you can make in advance and which need fresh ingredients that day.

Acorn Squash with Spiced Applesauce and Maple Drizzle Recipe

Prep Time: 8 Minutes
Style:American
Cook Time: 20 Minutes
Phase: Phase 3
Difficulty: Moderate

* Any adjustments made to the serving values will only update the ingredients of that recipe and not change the directions.
0.7g Protein, 3.3g Fat, 2.2g Fiber, 72.8kcalCalories, 9.7g Net Carbs.

INGREDIENTS
• 1 squash (4 inch diameter) Acorn Winter Squash
• 5 teaspoons unsalted butter stick
• 1/2 teaspoon salt
• 1/2 teaspoon Black Pepper
• 3/4 cup Applesauce (without added ascorbic acid, unsweetened, canned)
• 1/8 teaspoon Cinnamon
• 1 tablespoon Sugar free maple flavored Syrup

DIRECTIONS

1. Preheat oven to 350°F. Cut squash in half, remove seeds and then cut into 6 wedges.

2. Line a sheet pan with aluminum foil. Melt 1 tablespoon (3 teaspoons) butter and brush on squash; sprinkle with salt and pepper. Place on pan and bake until squash is fork tender, about 20 minutes.

3. In a small pot heat the applesauce, about 3 minutes. Stir in 2 teaspoons butter and cinnamon and cook 30 seconds more.

4. Serve squash with a dollop of applesauce mixture and a drizzle of syrup (about 1/2 teaspoon each).

COOKING TIP: Having a party? When planning your low carb spread, think about which dishes you can make in advance and which need fresh ingredients that day.

"Pasta" Salad with Pesto and Zucchini Ribbons Recipe

Prep Time: 10 Minutes
Style:Italian
Cook Time: 0 Minutes
Phase: Phase 2
Difficulty: Easy

* Any adjustments made to the serving values will only update the ingredients of that recipe and not change the directions.
4.2g Protein, 11.9g Fat, 1.8g Fiber, 150.6kcalCalories, 5.9g Net Carbs.

INGREDIENTS
• 2 cups zucchini noodles
• 10 each cherry or grape tomato
• 1/4 cup green bell pepper (chopped)
• 1/4 cup red bell pepper (chopped)
• 1/4 cup Red Onion (chopped)
• 16 each Kalamata Olives
• 1/4 cup, crumbled Feta Cheese
• 1 serving Basil Pesto
Ingredient notes: You will need ¼ cup of Atkins recipe for basil pesto, or you can use a premade pesto with no more than 2 net carbs for ¼ cup. We suggest using 2-inch long zucchini ribbons, or wavy ribbons, for

this recipe. Optionally, sprinkle with 2 tablespoons pine nuts for an extra 0.4 net carbs per serving.

DIRECTIONS
1. Fold together all ingredients in a medium bowl until evenly distributed and coated with pesto.

Kid friendly variation: Use 16 large black olives and 1-ounce mozzarella cheese instead of the Kalamata olives and feta cheese, and subtract 0.7 Net Carbs per serving.

Air Fryer Buffalo Cauliflower Recipe
Prep Time: 10 Minutes
Style:American
Cook Time: 5 Minutes
Phase: Phase 1
Difficulty: Moderate

* Any adjustments made to the serving values will only update the ingredients of that recipe and not change the directions.
32.3g Protein, 29.5g Fat, 2.6g Fiber, 419.4kcalCalories.

INGREDIENTS

- 5 servings Kroger Pork Rinds (1/2 ounce)
- 9 teaspoons Frank's Redhot Buffalo Wings Sauce
- 1 1/2 tablespoons Butter - Unsalted - Kroger Brand
- 2 1/4 servings Hot Sauce, Sriracha Hot Chili Sauce 1 teaspoon (5grams)
- 2/3 tablespoon Apple Cider Vinegar
- 1/4 head large (6-7" diameter) Cauliflower, raw
- 1 each Egg
- 1 1/2 ounces Maytag Blue Cheese

DIRECTIONS

1. Preheat your air fryer to 390°F for about 10 minutes while you are preparing the cauliflower.

2. Pulse 2.5 ounces of pork rinds in a food processor until they are broken down to a sand like texture, being careful not to over process into a paste. Measure out ¼ cup plus 2 tablespoons of the ground pork rinds into a large bowl. Add the hot wing sauce, melted butter, Sriracha, and vinegar to the pork rinds and stir until well combined. It will be a thick batter consistency.

3. In another medium to large bowl, whisk the egg until frothy.

4. Cut the cauliflower into florets, ensuring none are overly large, and place in the bowl with the egg. Toss to coat, ensuring that the egg gets into as many nooks and crannies in the cauliflower as possible. Then, one by one, coat each floret in the wing sauce batter, smoothing it onto the surface and into the nooks of the cauliflower so each floret is nicely coated.

5. Once the air fryer is preheated, arrange the cauliflower in a single layer in the basket. Cook for 5 minutes at 390°F. Remove from the fryer, sprinkle with the blue cheese and serve while hot.

Atkins Peanut Butter Granola Bar Parfait with Yogurt and Strawberries Recipe

Prep Time: 5 Minutes
Style:American
Cook Time: 0 Minutes
Phase: Phase 3
Difficulty: Easy

* Any adjustments made to the serving values will only update the ingredients of that recipe and not change the directions.
27.9g Protein, 11.3g Fat, 7.8g Fiber, 309.2kcalCalories, 13.6g Net Carbs.

INGREDIENTS
• 1/2 cup Greek Yogurt - Plain (Container)
• 5 large (1-3/8" diameter) Strawberries
• 1 each Atkins Peanut Butter Granola Bar

DIRECTIONS
This recipe uses one Atkins Peanut Butter Granola Bar that has been coarsely chopped. Another Atkins bar with 4g NC or less may be substituted as desired.

In a parfait glass, layer the chopped granola bar with the yogurt and diced or quartered strawberries.

COOKING TIP: Whether you're feeding a family or cooking for one, you can update the serving settings above to reveal the required amount of ingredients.

Atkins Yorkshire Pudding Recipe

Prep Time: 5 Minutes
Style:Other
Cook Time: 35 Minutes
Phase: Phase 3
Difficulty: Moderate

* Any adjustments made to the serving values will only update the ingredients of that recipe and not change the directions.
9.9g Protein, 12g Fat, 0.7g Fiber, 161.7kcalCalories, 3.4g Net Carbs.

INGREDIENTS
- 1/2 cup whole Grain Soy Flour
- 2 ounces vital wheat gluten
- 3 large eggs (whole)
- 1 cup whole milk
- 1 teaspoon salt
- 1/3 cup Canola Vegetable Oil
- 1 teaspoon baking powder (straight Phosphate, double acting)

DIRECTIONS
Torkshire Pudding is traditionally made with pan drippings from cooking meat. In this recipe oil is listed instead. Feel free to use pan drippings for a more flavorful pudding.

1. Preheat oven to 450° F.
2. Whisk together soy flour, gluten, eggs, milk and salt.
3. Pour drippings or oil into an 8-inch square baking dish, and place on center rack in oven for 5 minutes, until drippings or oil is smoking hot. Then add batter and bake 15 minutes.
4. Lower temperature to 350° F and bake for 15 to 20 minutes more, until lightly browned. Serve piping hot.

COOKING TIP: Having a party? When planning your low carb spread, think about which dishes you can make in advance and which need fresh ingredients that day.

Bagna Cauda Recipe

Prep Time: 5 Minutes
Style:Italian
Cook Time: 5 Minutes
Phase: Phase 1
Difficulty: Easy

* Any adjustments made to the serving values will only update the ingredients of that recipe and not change the directions.
1.3g Protein, 19.6g Fat, 0g Fiber, 180.2kcalCalories, 0.3gNet Carbs.

INGREDIENTS
• 1/2 cup extra virgin olive oil
• 1/4 cup unsalted butter stick
• 3 teaspoons garlic
• 8 each anchovy (Drained Solids In Oil, Canned)

DIRECTIONS

1. In a small saucepan, heat olive oil and butter over medium heat.

2. Add garlic and anchovies. Cook gently for 5 minutes, until garlic is fragrant (but not brown).

3. Add pepper to taste. Transfer to a hot pot or heated dish and serve with vegetables.

COOKING TIP: If you're serving as an appetizer, plate your dip with two or three different low carb snacks!

Baked Black Bass and Clams in Foil

Prep Time: 20 Minutes
Style:Asian
Cook Time: 10 Minutes
Phase: Phase 1
Difficulty: Moderate

* Any adjustments made to the serving values will only update the ingredients of that recipe and not change the directions.
39.3g Protein, 28.6g Fat, 0.6g Fiber, 435.2kcalCalories, 3.5g Net Carbs.

INGREDIENTS
- 1/2 cup extra virgin olive oil
- 4 tablespoons fish sauce
- 2 cloves garlic
- 2 tablespoons fresh lime juice
- 1/2 serving Crushed Red Pepper
- 1/2 cup sliced fennel bulk
- 1/2 cup chopped Celery
- 20 ounces Pacific cod (fish)
- 12 medium Clams

DIRECTIONS
The original recipe calls for black bass. Cod works wonderfully and easier to find. You could also use hake or another flakey white fish. Salmon also works well. Baking fish in foil has several advantages. It can be prepared ahead of time and there's no pan to clean or fishy odor in the kitchen. You also have total control of the temperature of the fish. This recipe also calls for kaffir lime leaves, they are available in Asian markets and some well-stocked supermarkets. Substitute with basil leaves or a little lime zest if you cannot find them. Additionally you will need 4 (6x8-inch) pieces of banana leaves or parchment paper.

1. Preheat oven to 375°F.

2. In a small bowl, mix together the olive oil, fish sauce, minced garlic, lime juice and red pepper flakes; set aside

3. Place pieces of foil on a clean, dry surface and top each with a banana leaf. Thinly slice the fennel and celery.

4. Divide the fennel and celery into four equal portions and place one portion of each on each banana leaf. Place 1 (5-ounce) bass filet, 3 clams and one-quarter of the kaffir lime leaves on the fennel and celery. Spoon the sauce over fish and vegetables.

5. Fold and crimp the edges of the foil to seal packets. Bake for 8-10 minutes, depending on the thickness of the fish.

6. Place each packet on a plate and serve. Be certain the clams are open before serving.

COOKING TIP: Whether you're feeding a family or cooking for one, you can update the serving settings above to reveal the required amount of ingredients.

Lemon Mousse Parfait with Lime Crema and Toasted Walnuts Recipe

Prep Time: 15 Minutes
Style:French
Cook Time: 20 Minutes
Phase: Phase 2
Difficulty: Difficult

* Any adjustments made to the serving values will only update the ingredients of that recipe and not change the directions.

9g Protein, 34.2g Fat, 1.5g Fiber, 362.3kcalCalories, 6.9g Net Carbs.

INGREDIENTS

• 1/4 cup chopped English Walnuts

• 9 tablespoons Fresh Lemon Juice

• 3 large eggs (whole)

• 3 large egg yolks

• 6 packets Stevia

• 2 tablespoons unsalted butter stick

• 3/4 cup Heavy Cream

• 5 tablespoons fresh lime juice

DIRECTIONS

This delicious dessert layers lemon curd, lime cream, and walnut for contrasts in color and texture. Use a zester, the fine side of a box grater or a micro plane to zest the lemons and limes. This recipe has been adjusted to the amount of zest and juice you will need. If you buy whole fruit then it will be 3 lemons and limes.

1. Preheat oven to 400° F. Place the walnuts on baking sheet and cook until brown, about 8 minutes, being careful not to burn.

2. Bring a large pot of water or a double boiler to a boil.

3. Zest the lemons and then juice them. Place zest and juice in a medium bowl or the top of a double boiler. Add the whole eggs and yolks. Place the bowl over the boiling water and turn heat down to low. With a hand mixer, whisk the eggs, yolks and lemon juice until mixture is creamy and doubles in volume. Remove from heat. Add

the butter and 4 packets sugar substitute to the bowl and allow the mixture to cool.

4. Place the cream in a mixing bowl. Zest and then juice the limes, as above. Add to the cream. Whisk the lime and cream mixture until soft peaks form. Add 2 packets of stevia.

5. In 4 parfait or martini glasses, layer first one-half of the lime crema, then one-third of the walnuts, followed by all the lemon curd. Next add another layer of walnuts and top them with the remaining lime crema.

COOKING TIP: We love the idea of customizing this recipe to make it your own! If you add any ingredients, just be sure to keep an eye on net carbs.

Braised Lamb Shanks with Spiced Quince Recipe

Prep Time: 35 Minutes
Style:Italian
Cook Time: 240 Minutes
Phase: Phase 3
Difficulty: Difficult

* Any adjustments made to the serving values will only update the ingredients of that recipe and not change the directions.

71.5g Protein, 52.5g Fat, 2.4g Fiber, 832kcalCalories, 11.5g Net Carbs.

INGREDIENTS

• 72 ounces lamb leg (Shank Half, Trimmed to 1/8" Fat, Choice Grade)

• 5 tablespoons canola vegetable oil

• 7 cups chicken broth, bouillon or consomme

• 2 cups sliced onions

• 10 cloves garlic

• 2 servings diced plum tomatoes

- 1/3 ounce thyme

- 1 1/4 each Bay Leaf

- 2 fruit without refuses Quinces

- 1/2 teaspoon Cinnamon

- 1/2 teaspoon whole black peppercorns

- 3 tablespoons peppermint (Mint)

DIRECTIONS

When I was growing up, my family rarely ate beef, but lamb was usually on the table, which may be why I tend to cook with it nowadays. The shank is one of my favorite cuts and is quite inexpensive. Although it takes a long time to cook, it has a delectably rich, buttery flavor and usually falls off the bone. Caramelizing the shanks before putting them in the oven further enhances the flavor of this dish. Lamb pairs well with fruit, and I usually braise in the fall and early winter when quince are in season. Looking like a cross between a pear and an apple, quince becomes sweet after cooking. Although the amount of meat may seem large, at least half of each shank is bone.

Note: You will need a 3-inch piece of cinnamon (or the 1/2 tsp ground cinnamon), 1 whole allspice berry and 2 whole cloves to make the quince sauce.

1. Preheat the oven to 325°F.

2. Season the lamb shanks with salt and pepper. Heat 3 tablespoons of canola oil in a large saute pan or skillet on high, and then add shanks. Sear for about 3-4 minutes on each side, or until golden-brown on all sides. Remove to a large braising pan.

3. Bring 1 cup of chicken broth to a boil, add to the saute pan and with the heat on low, deglaze the pan by scraping the remaining pieces of meat stuck to it with a whisk or spatula. Transfer to the braising pan with the shanks.

4. In a medium sauté pan, heat the remaining 2 tablespoons of canola oil and "sweat" the onions and garlic over medium-low heat, stirring occasionally, for about 12-14 minutes. The onions should be soft and translucent.

5. Add the tomato and 1 cup of chicken broth, bring to a simmer and then transfer

the mixture to the braising pan with the shanks.

6. Pour the remaining 4 cups of broth into the braising pan. Add the bay leaves and thyme. Cover with parchment paper or aluminum foil and a lid and place in the oven.

7. After the lamb has been cooking for about 3 hours, place the quince, 1 cup of chicken broth, cinnamon stick, peppercorns, allspice and cloves in a small sauce pot. Bring to a boil and then reduce heat and simmer for 45 minutes, or until tender. Remove the quince and keep warm. Discard the liquid and seasonings.

8. After about 4 hours of cooking, when the meat is tender and almost falling off the bone, remove the shanks from the oven and let them cool until they can be handled. (They should still be warm.) Remove the shanks from the pan, leaving the vegetables in the pan juices. Cover the shanks to keep them warm .

9. Place the braising pan on the top of the range and with two burners on medium-high, reduce the sauce by whisking it until it

is thick enough to coat a spoon for 45 minutes.

10. To serve, place one-sixth of the quince on the side of each plate with a shank next to it and lap the sauce over it. Top with mint.

COOKING TIP: Whether you're feeding a family or cooking for one, you can update the serving settings above to reveal the required amount of ingredients.

LOW CARB DESSERT RECIPES

Lemon Mousse Parfait with Lime Crema and Toasted Walnuts Recipe

Prep Time: 15 Minutes
Style:French
Cook Time: 20 Minutes
Phase: Phase 2
Difficulty: Difficult

* Any adjustments made to the serving values will only update the ingredients of that recipe and not change the directions.

9g Protein, 34.2g Fat, 1.5g Fiber, 362.3kcalCalories, 6.9g Net Carbs.

INGREDIENTS

- 1/4 cup chopped English Walnuts

- 9 tablespoons Fresh Lemon Juice

- 3 large eggs (whole)

- 3 large egg yolks

- 6 packets Stevia

- 2 tablespoons unsalted butter stick

- 3/4 cup Heavy Cream

- 5 tablespoons fresh lime juice

DIRECTIONS

This delicious dessert layers lemon curd, lime cream, and walnut for contrasts in color and texture. Use a zester, the fine side of a box grater or a micro plane to zest the lemons and limes. This recipe has been adjusted to the amount of zest and juice you will need. If you buy whole fruit then it will be 3 lemons and limes.

1. Preheat oven to 400° F. Place the walnuts on baking sheet and cook until brown, about 8 minutes, being careful not to burn.

2. Bring a large pot of water or a double boiler to a boil.

3. Zest the lemons and then juice them. Place zest and juice in a medium bowl or the top of a double boiler. Add the whole eggs and yolks. Place the bowl over the boiling water and turn heat down to low. With a hand mixer, whisk the eggs, yolks and lemon juice until mixture is creamy and doubles in volume. Remove from heat. Add the butter and 4 packets sugar substitute to the bowl and allow the mixture to cool.

4. Place the cream in a mixing bowl. Zest and then juice the limes, as above. Add to the cream. Whisk the lime and cream mixture until soft peaks form. Add 2 packets of stevia.

5. In 4 parfait or martini glasses, layer first one-half of the lime cream, then one-third of the walnuts, followed by all the lemon curd. Next add another layer of walnuts and top them with the remaining lime crema.

COOKING TIP: We love the idea of customizing this recipe to make it your own! If you add any ingredients, just be sure to keep an eye on net carbs.

Keto Almond Butter Protein Truffles

Prep Time: 55 Minutes
Style:American
Cook Time: 5 Minutes
Phase: Phase 2
Difficulty: Easy

* Any adjustments made to the serving values will only update the ingredients of that recipe and not change the directions.

3.3g Protein, 6.9g Fat, 2.3g Fiber, 82.1kcalCalories, 1.8g Net Carbs.

INGREDIENTS

• 6 tablespoons almond butter

• 6 tablespoon(s) coconut cream, canned unsweetened

• 1 scoop (1 scoop= 30 g) quest chocolate milkshake protein powder

• 3/4 teaspoon glucomannan, pure powder (1 tsp= 4 g)

• 1 dash salt

• 6 tablespoons chocolate chips, sugar free

• 1 teaspoon(s) coconut oil

DIRECTIONS

1. In a medium mixing bowl, mix the almond butter, coconut cream, and salt together until well combined. If both the almond butter and coconut cream are solid or cold, you may need to warm them either in the microwave (in a microwaves safe container) or over a pot of steaming water (in a heat proof bowl) to be able to completely incorporate.

2. Add the protein powder, glucomannan (or other finely ground fiber source), and mix until all the powder is worked in, and a smooth texture develops. The mixture will be slightly oily.

3. Line a baking sheet with parchment paper. Make 14 tablespoon mounds of the almond butter mixture on the parchment paper lined baking sheet and put into the freezer to cool for 10 minutes, or until chilled enough to form into a ball. Form into balls and freeze until well set, another 20 minutes.

4. While the balls are cooling, use a double boiler (or in a medium heat proof bowl over a small saucepan with about 1-inch simmering water) to melt the chocolate chips and coconut oil together, stirring until fully melted and uniform texture. Keep warm until the balls are well cooled.

5. Remove the balls from the freezer and, one at a time, roll in the melted chocolate to coat. Place each coated truffle back on the parchment paper and refrigerate until the chocolate has hardened, about 10 minutes. Store in an airtight container in the refrigerator for up to one week. One truffle is one serving.

COOKING TIP: Try adding diced freeze dried strawberries as a variation. Adding in 1-2 freeze dried strawberry slices won't change the NC of this naturally keto and low carb recipe enough to worry about so just enjoy!

Apricot-Apple Cloud Recipe

Prep Time: 65 Minutes
Style:American
Cook Time: 0 Minutes
Phase: Phase 3
Difficulty: Easy

* Any adjustments made to the serving values will only update the ingredients of that recipe and not change the directions.
1.4g Protein, 22.2g Fat, 1.4g Fiber, 241.7kcalCalories, 9.8g Net Carbs.

INGREDIENTS
• 1 1/2 cups heavy cream
• 2 tablespoons sucralose based sweetener (Sugar Substitute)
• 16 ounces Baby Food Applesauce and Apricots

DIRECTIONS
This no-cook dessert uses a surprise ingredient: baby food. Be sure to use a product without added sugar and to allow at least an hour to chill the dessert.

1. With an electric mixer on medium, beat cream and sugar substitute until medium-firm peaks form.

2. Gently fold in baby food (you will need 16 oz or four 4 oz jars).

3. Divide among 6 dessert glasses and chill at least 1 hour before serving.

COOKING TIP: We love the idea of customizing this recipe to make it your own! If you add any ingredients, just be sure to keep an eye on net carbs.

Atkins Cinnamon Pie Crust Recipe

Prep Time: 10 Minutes
Style:American
Cook Time: 0 Minutes
Phase: Phase 3
Difficulty: Easy

* Any adjustments made to the serving values will only update the ingredients of that recipe and not change the directions.
9g Protein, 13.5g Fat, 1.6g Fiber, 168.4kcalCalories, 2.4g Net Carbs

INGREDIENTS
- 1/4 teaspoon salt
- 1 teaspoon sucralose based sweetener (sugar substitute)
- 1 teaspoon cinnamon
- 1/2 cup unsalted butter stick
- 2 tablespoons tap water
- 3 3/4 servings Atkins Flour Mix

DIRECTIONS
Use the Atkins recipe to make Atkins Flour Mix. You will need 1 1/4 cups to make one pie crust.

1. Pulse the baking mix, salt, sugar substitute, and cinnamon in a food processor to incorporate; add butter and pulse until mixture resembles a coarse meal, about 30 seconds. Pulse in water until dough just comes together, about 30 seconds (add up to 1 more tablespoon if necessary).

2. Transfer dough to a sheet of plastic wrap; form into a disk about 6 inches in diameter. Wrap tightly in plastic; refrigerate until firm, about 30 minutes.

3. Roll and bake as directed in pie recipe. Makes 1 pie crust.

Find this recipe and more in the New Atkins For a New You Cookbook!

COOKING TIP: We love the idea of customizing this recipe to make it your own! If you add any ingredients, just be sure to keep an eye on net carbs.

Berries with Chocolate Ganache Recipe

Prep Time: 10 Minutes
Style:French
Cook Time: 5 Minutes
Phase: Phase 2
Difficulty: Easy

* Any adjustments made to the serving values will only update the ingredients of that recipe and not change the directions.
4g Protein, 17.6g Fat, 8.1g Fiber, 286.3kcalCalories, 9.5g Net Carbs.

INGREDIENTS
- 8 ounces strawberries
- 2 cups red raspberries
- 2 cups fresh blueberries
- 8 ounces sugar free chocolate chips
- 1/3 cup heavy cream
- 1/2 teaspoon vanilla extract

DIRECTIONS
1. Combine fruit and place into 6 dessert bowls.
2. In a small saucepan over low heat, heat chocolate and cream until just melted (this can be done in a microwave for 30 seconds at a time. Be careful not to overheat and burn the chocolate). Add vanilla and stir until smooth.
3. Cool slightly and drizzle sauce over fruit just before serving.

COOKING TIP: We love the idea of customizing this recipe to make it your own! If you add any ingredients, just be sure to keep an eye on net carbs.

Blackberry-Orange Sorbet Recipe

Prep Time: 240 Minutes
Style:American
Cook Time: 20 Minutes
Phase: Phase 3
Difficulty: Easy

* Any adjustments made to the serving values will only update the ingredients of that recipe and not change the directions.
3.6g Protein, 1.6g Fat, 4.3g Fiber, 75.9kcalCalories, 8.5g Net Carbs.

INGREDIENTS
• 2 1/4 cups blackberries
• 1 teaspoon orange zest
• 1 cup buttermilk (Reduced Fat, Cultured)
• 1/3 cup sucralose based sweetener (Sugar Substitute)

DIRECTIONS
1. In a medium saucepan, bring blackberries, sugar substitute, 2 tablespoons water, and orange zest to a boil. Reduce heat and simmer, covered, for 15 minutes, stirring occasionally, until berries break down. Cool quickly by placing in a bowl sitting in

another larger bowl filled with an ice water bath.

2. Place cooled berry mixture in a food processor. Process until smooth. Press through a fine strainer into a bowl. Stir in buttermilk. Chill in refrigerator 1 hour or until cold.

3. Pour into an ice-cream maker and run according to manufacturer's directions. Transfer to a bowl and freeze 2 to 3 hours before serving. 1 serving is about 1/2 cup.

COOKING TIP: We love the idea of customizing this recipe to make it your own! If you add any ingredients, just be sure to keep an eye on net carbs.

Blueberry and Almond Protein Mousse Recipe

Prep Time: 15 Minutes
Style: American
Cook Time: 0 Minutes
Phase: Phase 2
Difficulty: Easy

* Any adjustments made to the serving values will only update the ingredients of that recipe and not change the directions.
4.9g Protein, 20.4g Fat, 1.9g Fiber, 222.7kcalCalories, 5.1g Net Carbs

INGREDIENTS
• 4 tablespoons cream cheese, original
• 28 grams Atkins vanilla protein powder
• 1 cup, fluid (yields 2 cups whipped) heavy whipping cream
• 1/3 teaspoon almond extract
• 1 cup blueberries, fresh
• 1/4 cup sliced almonds

DIRECTIONS

1. With an electric mixer blend together the softened cream cheese and protein powder until smooth. Set aside.

2. In a separate bowl whip the heavy cream with the almond extract until doubled in volume.

3. Gently add 1/3 of the whipped cream to the cream cheese mixture blending by hand until smooth. Add another 3rd of the whipped cream folding it into the mixture until well blended. Add the final 3rd of the whipped cream, folding until fully incorporated. Divide into 6 serving bowls, cover with plastic wrap and refrigerate until ready to serve.

4. To toast the almonds, place them on a sheet pan and toast for 3-5 minutes at 350°F. Sprinkle each bowl with blueberries and sliced almonds before serving.

COOKING TIP: We love the idea of customizing this recipe to make it your own! If you add any ingredients, just be sure to keep an eye on net carbs.

Cafe Caramel Panna Cotta

Prep Time: 5 Minutes
Style:American
Cook Time: 10 Minutes
Phase: Phase 2
Difficulty: Easy

* Any adjustments made to the serving values will only update the ingredients of that recipe and not change the directions.
4.7g Protein, 23.5g Fat, 0.2g Fiber, 237.8kcalCalories, 2.1g Net Carbs.

INGREDIENTS
- 1 envelope gelatin, unsweetened
- 2 tablespoons tap water
- 1 1/2 cups Heavy Cream, liquid
- 1 each Atkins café caramel shake
- 3 tablespoons confectioners (powdered) erythritol
- 5 drops liquid stevia drops
- 1 teaspoon vanilla extract

Ingredient note: We recommend using English Toffee flavored liquid stevia drops for this recipe.

DIRECTIONS

1. In a cup, sprinkle the gelatin onto the water and set aside.

2. In a small saucepan, whisk together the cream, shake, sweeteners and vanilla. Warm over medium heat, stirring occasionally, until just starting to simmer, about 10 minutes.

3. Remove from heat, and whisk in the gelatin until dissolved. Fill 6 ramekins with ½ cup of the liquid, cover with plastic wrap, and refrigerate for at least 3 hours or until the gelatin is set.

OPTIONAL: serve with a dollop of whipped cream (1 tablespoon adds .021 net carbs), or a teaspoon of sugar free caramel syrup (does not add net carbs).

VARIATIONS: We developed this recipe using the Café Caramel shake, but you could substitute any other shake for a wealth of flavor options.

LOW CARB BEVERAGE RECIPES

Almond-Pineapple Smoothie Recipe

Prep Time: 5 Minutes
Style: American
Cook Time: Minutes
Phase: Phase 3
Difficulty: Easy

* Any adjustments made to the serving values will only update the ingredients of that recipe and not change the directions.
10.7g Protein, 17.3g Fat, 3.9g Fiber, 275.7kcalCalories, 16.1g Net Carbs.

INGREDIENTS
• 1/2 cup (8 fluid ounces) plain yogurt (whole milk)
• 2 1/2 ounces pineapple
• 20 each wholes blanched & slivered almonds
• 1/2 cup pure almond milk - unsweetened original

DIRECTIONS

Feel free to substitute other fruits or nuts for the pineapple and/or almonds (about 20 whole almonds, 3 Tbsp slivered). Be sure to use fresh pineapple in this smoothie. Canned pineapple is swimming in sugar.

Combine the yogurt, pineapple, almonds and almond milk in a blender and purée until smooth and creamy.

COOKING TIP: Whether you're feeding a family or cooking for one, you can update the serving settings above to reveal the required amount of ingredients.

Atkins Chocolate Slushies Recipe

Prep Time: 5 Minutes
Style: American
Cook Time: 10 Minutes
Phase: Phase 1
Difficulty: Easy

* Any adjustments made to the serving values will only update the ingredients of that recipe and not change the directions.
2.8g Protein, 22.4g Fat, 1.9g Fiber, 229.5kcalCalories, 6.4g Net Carbs.

INGREDIENTS
• 1 cup Heavy Cream
• 1/2 cup tap water
• 2 tablespoons cocoa powder (unsweetened)
• 1/2 cup Sugar Free Chocolate Syrup
• 1 teaspoon vanilla extract

DIRECTIONS
1. In a medium saucepan combine cream, water, cocoa powder and 1/2 cup unsweetened chocolate syrup.
2. Bring to a boil over medium heat. Reduce heat to low; cook, stirring occasionally, 5 minutes. Remove from heat and stir in vanilla.

3. Pour mixture into two ice cube trays. Freeze 2 hours.

4. Before serving transfer cubes into a food processor. Pulse until mixture is finely chopped and slushy.

COOKING TIP: Why not have friends over to enjoy this drink! Update the serving settings above to reveal the required amount of ingredients you'll need.

Almond Raspberry Smoothie Recipe

Prep Time: 5 Minutes
Style: American
Cook Time: Minutes
Phase: Phase 2
Difficulty: Easy

* Any adjustments made to the serving values will only update the ingredients of that recipe and not change the directions.
18.2g Protein, 13.7g Fat, 6.9g Fiber, 259.4kcalCalories, 10.3g Net Carbs.

INGREDIENTS
- 4 ounces Greek Yogurt - Plain (Container)
- 1/2 cup Red Raspberries
- 20 each wholes Blanched & Slivered almonds
- 1/2 cup pure almond milk - unsweetened original

DIRECTIONS
Feel free to come up with your own combination of other berries and nuts for this protein-packed smoothie. If you use frozen raspberries, make sure they contain no added sugar.

Combine the yogurt, raspberries, almonds and almond milk in a blender and purée until smooth and creamy.

COOKING TIP: Whether you're feeding a family or cooking for one, you can update the serving settings above to reveal the required amount of ingredients.

Avocado Gazpacho Smoothie Recipe

Prep Time: 5 Minutes
Style: Mexican
Cook Time: 0 Minutes
Phase: Phase 1
Difficulty: Easy

* Any adjustments made to the serving values will only update the ingredients of that recipe and not change the directions.
9.1g Protein, 38.2g Fat, 11.9g Fiber, 419.5kcalCalories, 4.7g Net Carbs.

 INGREDIENTS
• 1 fruit without skin and seed California Avocado
• 1 ounce goat cheese (Soft)
• 1 tablespoon heavy cream
• 2 teaspoons fresh lime juice
• 1/8 teaspoon salt
• 1 cup Tap water
• 2 teaspoons chopped chives

DIRECTIONS

1. Place cut-up avocado in a blender. Add remaining ingredients, and blend until smooth. If needed, add additional water, 1 tablespoon at a time, to reach desired consistency.

2. Pour into a tall glass, and garnish with chives and a reserved slice of avocado, if desired. Serve immediately.

COOKING TIP: Whether you're feeding a family or cooking for one, you can update the serving settings above to reveal the required amount of ingredients.

Hazelnut Hot Chocolate Recipe

Prep Time: 5 Minutes
Style: American
Cook Time: 2 Minutes
Phase: Phase 1
Difficulty: Easy

* Any adjustments made to the serving values will only update the ingredients of that recipe and not change the directions.
17.9g Protein, 20.9g Fat, 5.9g Fiber, 286.1kcalCalories, 3.5g Net Carbs.

INGREDIENTS
• 14 nuts Hazelnuts
• 1/4 teaspoon vanilla extract
• 1 each Atkins Dark Chocolate Royale Shake

DIRECTIONS

1. Place chopped hazelnuts, vanilla (can substitute hazelnut extract for more hazelnut flavor) and 1/3 of the shake into a blender and blend on high until creamy and all the hazelnuts have been broken down; about 30 seconds. Add the remaining shake and blend until smooth.

2. Pour into a sauce pan and heat gently over medium heat while stirring until hot but not boiling. Pour into a mug and enjoy with a sprinkle of ground cinnamon.

NOTE: This may also be heated in a microwave but do so at 30 second intervals as it will foam with heating and may overflow your cup.

COOKING TIP: We love the idea of customizing this recipe to make it your own! If you add any ingredients, just be sure to keep an eye on net carbs.

Gin Fizz Recipe

Prep Time: 0 Minutes
Style: American
Cook Time: 0 Minutes
Phase: Phase 2
Difficulty: Easy

* Any adjustments made to the serving values will only update the ingredients of that recipe and not change the directions.
4.6g Protein, 16.6g Fat, 0.1g Fiber, 252.2kcalCalories, 3.3g Net Carbs.

INGREDIENTS
- 1 fluid ounce (no ice) Gin
- 1 wedge lime juice
- 1 wedge Lemon juice
- 1/2 teaspoon orange zest
- 1 packet no calorie sweetener packets
- 1 large white egg
- 3 tablespoons Heavy Cream
- 1/4 serving Original Seltzer Water (Can)

DIRECTIONS

For Cocktail: Shake all except seltzer in a cocktail mixer with ice. Strain into a cocktail glass, top off with seltzer and garnish with ground cinnamon and freshly grated nutmeg. Note that you will need about 1 tsp each of the lemon and lime juice.

It is best to use pasteurized eggs for this recipe. They can be hard to find except during the holiday months.

To pasteurze: place room temperature large eggs in a small saucepan covered with cold water. (Be sure they are at room temperature otherwise they will not get warm enough to pasteurize through to the yolk.) Place pan on the stove and cook over medium heat. Bring water to 140°F (but not higher than 145°F). It is best to use a thermometer but if you don't have a thermometer, 150° F is right about the time bubbles begin forming on the bottom of the pan. Allow the eggs to stay at that temperature for 3 minutes then quickly remove from the pan and cool under coldwater. Refrigerate until ready to use.

COOKING TIP: Why not have friends over to enjoy this drink? Update the serving settings above to reveal the required amount of ingredients you'll need.

Frozen Mocha Slushie Recipe

Prep Time: 5 Minutes
Style: American
Cook Time: 2 Minutes
Phase: Phase 1
Difficulty: Easy

* Any adjustments made to the serving values will only update the ingredients of that recipe and not change the directions.
2.3g Protein, 22.8g Fat, 1.8g Fiber, 225.7kcalCalories, 4.9g Net Carbs.

INGREDIENTS
• 4 fluid ounces decaffeinated coffee
• 3 tablespoons sugar-free chocolate syrup, Hershey's
• 2 tablespoons cocoa powder (Unsweetened)
• 2 teaspoons No Calorie Sweetener
• 1/2 cup Heavy Cream

DIRECTIONS

This recipe is a too high in NC for phase 1 but if you make only half a serving as a dessert or treat it is acceptable.

1. In a small saucepan over medium heat, stir together the coffee, chocolate syrup and cocoa powder. Stir until cocoa has dissolved, about 2 minutes. Cool slightly.

2. Transfer to a blender. Add sugar substitute and cream; blend until combined. Add 12 to 14 ice cubes in batches; blending until frothy.

COOKING TIP: Why not have friends over to enjoy this drink? Update the serving settings above to reveal the required amount of ingredients you'll need.

Cinnamon Spiced Coconut-Vanilla Protein Shake Recipe

Prep Time: 5 Minutes
Style: American
Cook Time: 0 Minutes
Phase: Phase 1
Difficulty: Easy

* Any adjustments made to the serving values will only update the ingredients of that recipe and not change the directions.
25g Protein, 4.5g Fat, 1.6g Fiber, 164.1kcalCalories, 2.6g Net Carbs.

INGREDIENTS
• 3 ice cubes (3/4 fluid ounce) water
• 1 cup Coconut milk unsweetened
• 1 ounce or scoop vanilla whey protein
• 1/2 teaspoon cinnamon
• 1/2 teaspoon vanilla extract

DIRECTIONS
1. Combine all ingredients in a blender and blend until smooth. If your protein powder does not have stevia or another granulated sugar substitute consider adding up to 1 teaspoon (add .5g NC) of sucralose (add .5g NC to the total grams of NC) or xylitol (no

additional g NC need to be added for xylitol or additional stevia).

COOKING TIP: Whether you're feeding a family or cooking for one, you can update the serving settings above to reveal the required amount of ingredients.

Extra-Creamy Strawberry Shake Recipe

Prep Time: 5 Minutes
Style: American
Cook Time: 0 Minutes
Phase: Phase 2
Difficulty: Easy

* Any adjustments made to the serving values will only update the ingredients of that recipe and not change the directions.
26.5g Protein, 22.1g Fat, 0.7g Fiber, 336.2kcalCalories, 5.9g Net Carbs.

INGREDIENTS
- 6 medium (1-1/4" diameter) Strawberries
- 2 scoops strawberry whey protein
- 1/2 cup heavy cream
- 1 teaspoon vanilla extract
- 2 cups tap water
- 2 individual packets sucralose based sweetener (sugar substitute)

DIRECTIONS
1. Place strawberries, protein powder, cream, vanilla, water, and sugar substitute in a blender and blend at high speed until very smooth.

COOKING TIP: Whether you're feeding a family or cooking for one, you can update the serving settings above to reveal the required amount of ingredients.

CPSIA information can be obtained
at www.ICGtesting.com
Printed in the USA
LVHW050344291220
675195LV00008B/258

9 781801 270045